fermented
probiotic drinks
at home

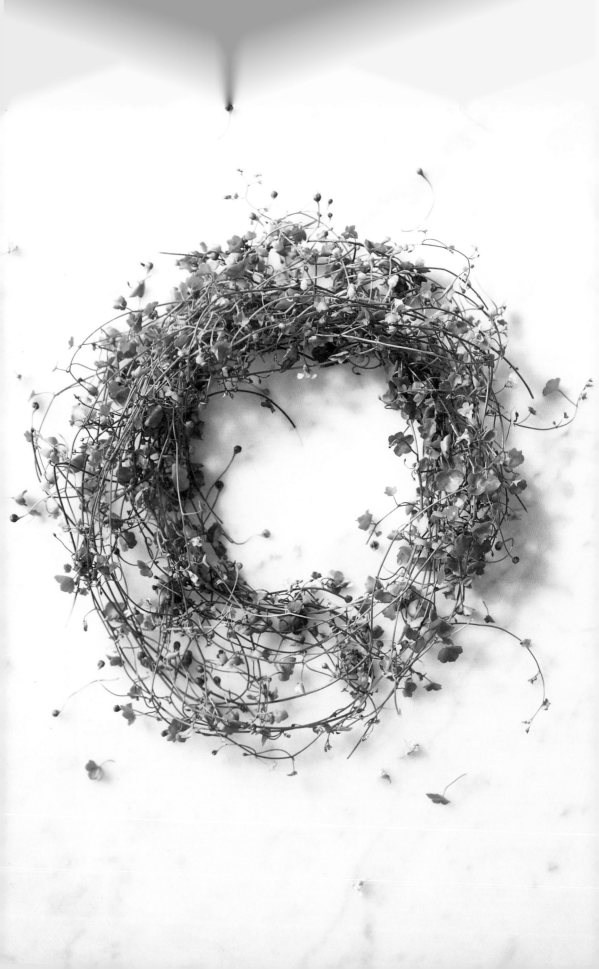

fermented
probiotic drinks
at home

MAKE YOUR OWN
Kombucha, Kefir, Ginger Bug, Jun,
Pineapple Tepache, Honey Mead,
Beet Kvass & More

Felicity Evans

THE EXPERIMENT

NEW YORK

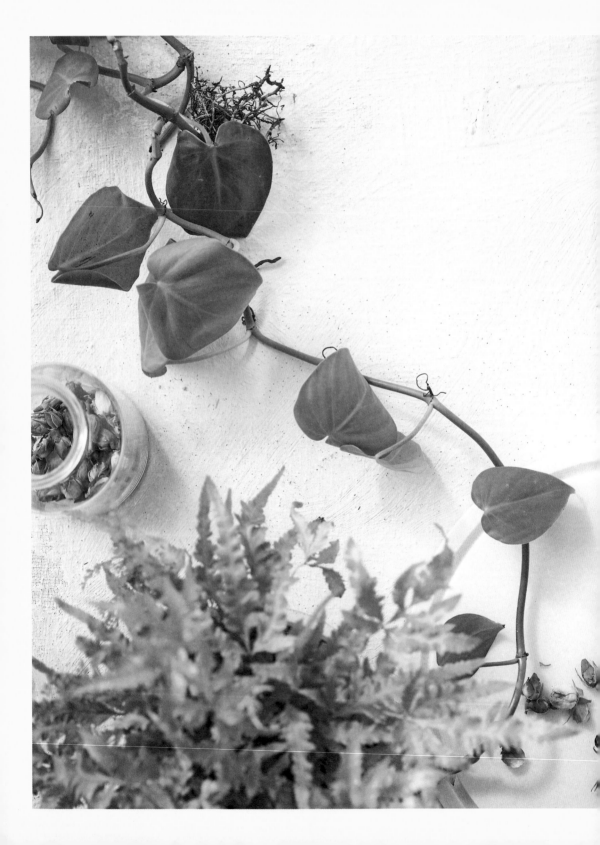

CONTENTS

PREFACE

Probiotic drinks have ancient roots but they are a relative newcomer to the healthy drinks menu. They provide an amazing source of energy, can aid in detoxification and boost overall health, and their true benefits are only just coming to light. The brilliant news is that you can create these elixirs in your kitchen.

My journey with fermentation and probiotic drinks has had an incredible impact on both my health and my family life. When I first started making probiotic drinks at home, I did so purely out of necessity. Having traveled the world with my husband on many amazing adventures, I battled with a string of diseases, including glandular fever, chronic fatigue and malaria. These left me bedridden and lethargic, and I was propped up by antibiotics.

After the birth of my second daughter, I suffered long-term chronic mastitis, requiring many rounds of antibiotics, and my overall health went well and truly downhill. I started to ask questions: What grinch stole my mojo? Why I am so unwell when I eat so well? Will I ever feel normal again? And, most crucially, what can I do to get my energy back?

I recalled an encounter with Guatemalan locals six years earlier where I tasted a sacred probiotic beverage – water kefir – known for its life-giving properties. It was fresh, slightly sparkling and not too sweet. And it made me feel amazing.

So, with a young baby strapped to my chest and a toddler at my heels, I began my kitchen fermentation trials, hoping to re-create that magical probiotic elixir I had been blessed to receive all those years ago. These early trials gave me an interesting taste of the highs and lows of fermentation, but overall the highs outweighed the lows. After a slow and steady start, my energy soon returned and I saw the positive effects on my health.

It was incredible to see my health being transformed from day to day. I fell in love with the fermentation process – the delight in hearing the bubbling and hissing, tasting the beautiful elixirs, the fizz on the tongue and the acidic zing – transforming the spices, herbs and berries into life-giving probiotic drinks through sheer alchemy. It was an exciting gateway into a new world.

Affectionately dubbed "Queen Alchemist," I realized I had a knack for the fermentation process, particularly with water kefir. I was invited to stock my water kefirs in a local health food store and from there Imbibe Living, my company, was born.

Fermentation is so special to me. It's like finding diamond treasures in your own home that you never knew existed. Through patience, trial and error, and the utmost of respect for ancient cultures, I've taught myself fermentation techniques and created these recipes that I'm delighted to share with you. By mixing some water, sugar and fresh ginger together you can create a refreshing, probiotic-rich, old-fashioned ginger beer. By stirring some honey and water together you can make your very own alcoholic honey mead.

Through fermentation, you create a happy home for your gut microbes, the foundation of good health and wellness. And there's a meditative rhythm to fermentation that I find satisfying to the soul. Like the seasons, you can lean in, embrace and connect to it.

So carve out the time, start simple, connect to your senses and watch a whole new world open up. A pinch of patience, a spoonful of curiosity and a willingness to learn are all you need to be on your way.

Fermentation has given me more than kitchen skills. It has given me a community, a way of life and a family tradition that I am proud to hand down to my children. I'm so excited to have the opportunity to inspire you to start your own home fermentation journey. Join me in transforming your health, one delicious drink at a time.

Felicity Evans
imbibeliving.com

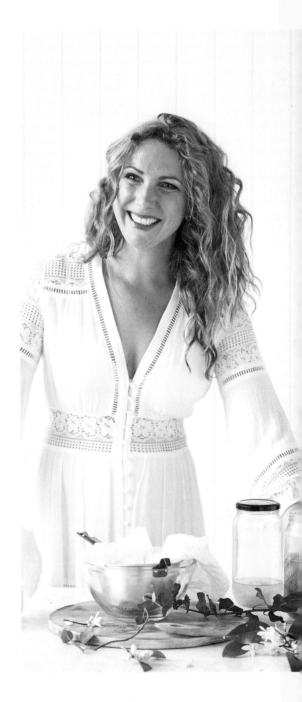

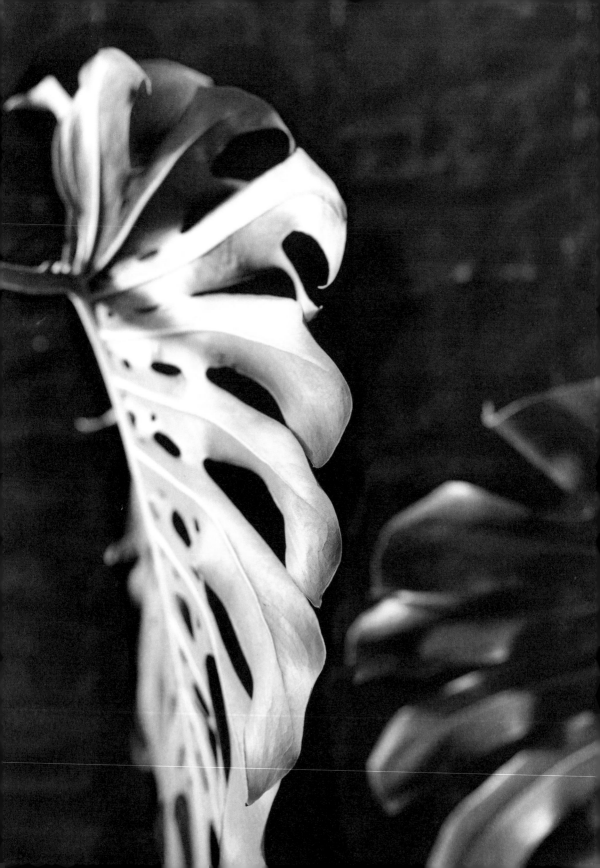

GOOD HEALTH STARTS IN THE GUT

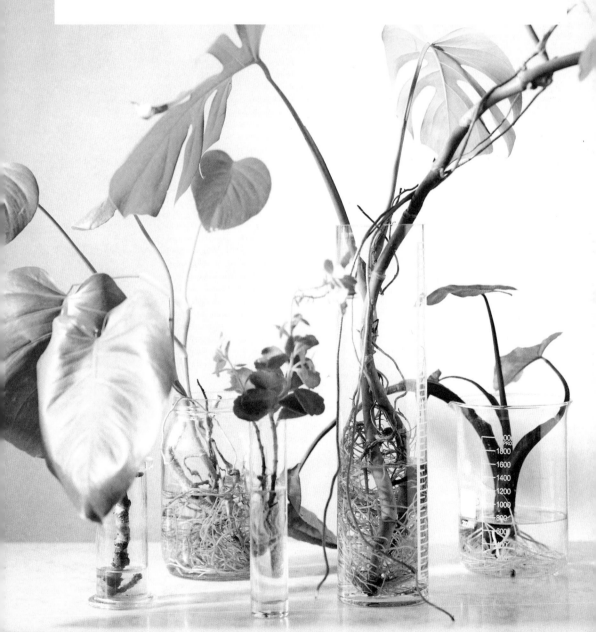

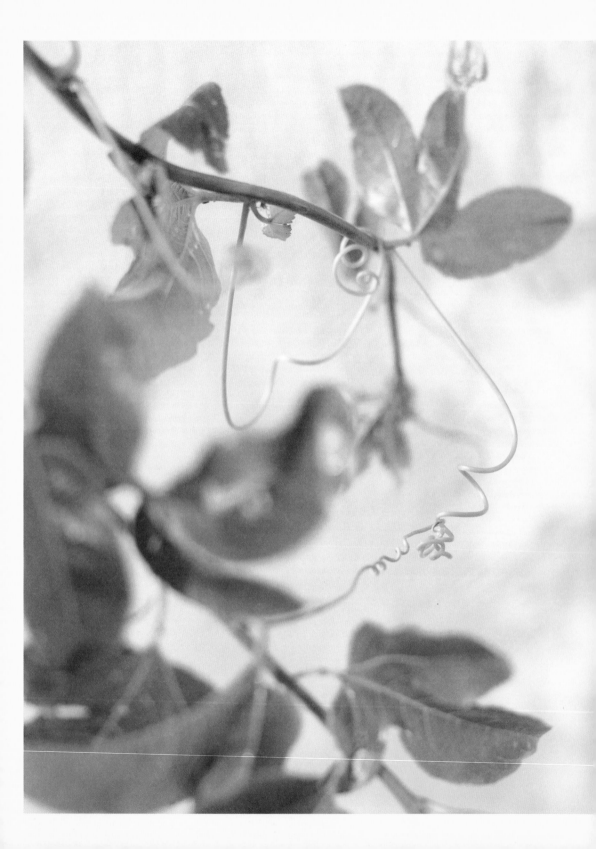

INTRODUCTION

The topic of probiotics and gut health is a vast and complex subject. Here is a small insight into this fascinating universe.

WHAT ARE PROBIOTICS?

Probiotic means "for life" (*pro* means "for" and *biotic* means "relating to life"). Probiotics are the good bacteria that are one of the keys to overall wellness. They add "good" bacteria to your gut to outweigh the "bad" bacteria. All the recipes in this book are aimed at giving you living probiotics to enhance your gut health, which enhances your overall wellness.

Probiotics have a varied role in the digestive system. They:
* assist with the manufacture of B vitamins
* protect against external toxins
* improve the efficiency of the gastrointestinal tract
* boost the immune system
* improve bowel function
* help to digest and absorb the nutrients from food.

WHAT ARE PREBIOTICS?

Prebiotics are indigestible fiber that serves as food for the probiotics in the gut, allowing them to thrive. Examples of prebiotics are:
* artichoke
* dandelion
* garlic
* onion
* leek
* corn
* cabbage.

probiotics

Good bacteria that help digest and absorb the nutrients from your food

prebiotics

Indigestible fiber that feeds the probiotics in your gut

HOW GUT HEALTH BECOMES UNBALANCED

* Chemicals in food, water and air
* Poor diet and food choices, including sugar, gluten and preservatives in processed foods
* Stress
* Medications, including antibiotics

HOW DO WE OBTAIN "GOOD" BACTERIA?

* By consuming fermented foods and drinks
* By taking probiotic dietary supplements
* By feeding the probiotics contained in the gut with prebiotics in the form of fiber-rich foods

THE GUT: THE CORNERSTONE OF GOOD HEALTH

The gut is the king and queen of the body systems and needs to be nurtured by living probiotics and nourishing foods to keep it functioning optimally. All the recipes in this book are designed to do just that.

In addition to processing and digesting the nutrients from our food, and being responsible for effective elimination, the gut is integral to other vital body functions. It's home to around 80 percent of the immune system and is also where many hormones and neurons are made and metabolized. Enzymes and nutrients that are important for vitality are also made and housed in the gut. Pathogens like bad bacteria and viruses can be overcome with a strong gut, which in turn should lead to fewer illnesses.

YOUR GUT: THE CORNERSTONE OF GOOD HEALTH IN THREE MAIN WAYS

DIGESTION

IMMUNITY

EMOTIONAL WELL-BEING

Increasing evidence shows that an imbalance of gut bacteria can be implicated in a whole host of diseases and conditions like asthma, allergies, arthritis and obesity.

Having a robust gut means that nutrients from food are better absorbed and utilized by the body. This leads to glowing skin, stronger hair and nails, and increased energy.

Probiotics contribute to good gut health, which leads to good digestion, good immunity and good emotional well-being. The bottom line: if you want excellent overall health, focus on probiotics, good nutrition, the integrity of your gut and moderate daily exercise, and the rest should follow.

DIGESTION

Good health begins in the gut. The old adage "you are what you eat" is only partly true; "you are what you absorb" would be a more accurate statement. You could eat the most nutritious diet possible, but if your gut microbiota is weak and can't properly digest and absorb nutrients it won't do you much good. That's why having good digestion is one of the keys to having great overall health, and why improving the function of your digestive system will help improve your well-being.

It could be said that digestion actually begins in the mind, with how you feel about foods and drinks and your relationship to eating and drinking.

Physical digestion is the breakdown and absorption of nutrients from food, which starts in the mouth and continues through the gut. If it was laid out end to end, the digestive system would be around 30 feet (9 meters) long.

We need a regular intake of probiotics to help digest and absorb the nutrients from the food we eat, as well as to increase the number of good bacteria that are essential for good health. Prebiotics also play an important role because they feed the probiotics.

Whether we realize it or not, we damage our digestive system daily, through medications, environmental toxins, food choices and lifestyle. Consuming probiotic drinks is a delicious way to help repair and strengthen the digestive system. The fermentation process that's used to produce probiotic drinks increases the nutrient profile of the ingredients they contain and makes them much more absorbable.

THE MICROBIOTA

Your body is made up of trillions of bacteria that live in and on you. The name of this complex and vast group of bacteria is the microbiota. Almost all microbiota live in your gastrointestinal tract. Like fingerprints, every person has his or her own unique microbiota and there are countless strains of bacteria that make up your microbiota. That's why it's a good idea to consume a variety of probiotic strains in the form of different fermented foods and drinks to add to this diversity. The "microbiome" is the genetic information contained in the microbiota.

IMMUNITY

The gut houses around 80 percent of your immune cells, so it's a good idea to first work on your gut health in order to enhance your immunity. Think of the immune cells as lab technicians in white coats, interviewing suspects to see whether they are good or bad, and calling in reinforcements if any of the suspects need to be shown the door.

Because the gut is an easy entry point for dangerous pathogens, your digestive system acts as a barrier between you and the outside world. This barrier has a diverse range of gut flora that helps protect against invaders. There is also an intestinal mucus layer that lines the gut, forming another barrier to keep invaders out of your body. Probiotics and prebiotics help to stimulate the production of this mucus layer.

Even if you are generally healthy, taking living probiotics in the form of fermented foods and drinks is an important step in increasing and maintaining the integrity of your gut and therefore boosting your immunity.

EMOTIONAL WELL-BEING

Your gut is responsible for around 80 to 90 percent of the production of serotonin, the amazing feel-good hormone that we all love. This is why the gut is sometimes called "the second brain." When the "good" gut bacteria are overtaken by the "bad" bacteria, serotonin production and other chemical reactions in your body are impeded.

You also have around 500 million nerve cells and around 100 million neurons in your intestines, which communicate with your brain via the vagus nerve that connects the brain to the abdomen.

There are two nervous systems in the body:
* **central nervous system:** your brain and spinal cord
* **enteric nervous system:** a mesh-like system of neurons controlling your gastrointestinal tract and responsible for neurotransmitters, hormone production and peristalsis.

THE VAGUS NERVE

The central and enteric nervous systems are linked by a superhighway called the vagus nerve, an incredible nerve that connects the brain to the abdomen.

Exercise the efficiency of the vagus nerve in the following simple ways.
1. Practice loud singing and gargling for 30 seconds each day.
2. Meditate daily to help calm the nervous system and encourage good digestion.
3. Focus on deep, long, slow breathing to settle the nervous system.

METHODS OF
FERMENTATION

There are two main styles of fermentation used to create probiotic drinks: **Cultured fermentation** and **Wild fermentation**.

CULTURED FERMENTATION

This relies on an acquired starter culture – a symbiotic colony of bacteria and yeasts or "SCOBY" – to start the fermentation process. You can source starter cultures online.

CULTURED FERMENTATION DRINKS

Water kefir
A fizzy, tangy, water-based probiotic drink that uses water kefir culture to ferment sugar water

Coconut water kefir
A fizzy, tangy, coconut water–based probiotic drink that uses water kefir culture to ferment coconut water

Milk kefir
A slightly effervescent, sour, milk-based probiotic drink that uses milk kefir culture to ferment whole milk or nut milks

Kombucha
A fermented tea tonic, made by using a kombucha SCOBY to ferment sweetened green, black or herbal tea

Jun
A fermented green tea and honey drink, made by using a Jun SCOBY to ferment green tea and honey

WILD FERMENTATION

This is spontaneous and relies on the naturally occurring yeasts and bacteria found in the air and on the skins of fruits, vegetables and roots to start the fermentation process.

WILD FERMENTATION DRINKS

Beet kvass
A sour beet drink that relies on wild yeasts to convert beets and water into a probiotic beet tonic

Pineapple tepache
A sweet, highly effervescent probiotic drink made by fermenting pineapple skins, sugar and water

Ginger bug
A starter culture used to make ginger beer and root beer; ginger bug is made by combining water, ginger and sugar and allowing the wild yeasts to transform the sugars into a bubbly probiotic mixture

Honey mead
A combination of honey and water that is stirred regularly, attracting wild yeasts to convert the sugars into probiotics

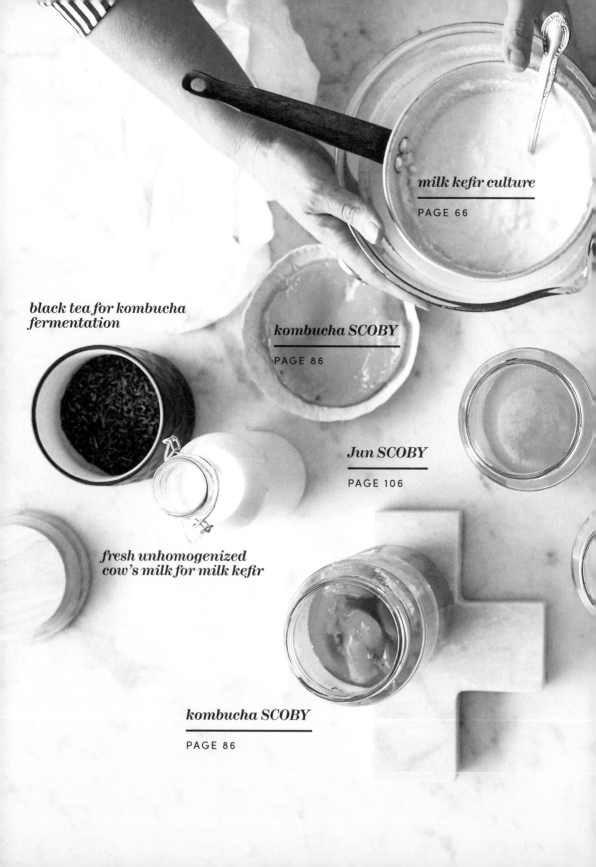

milk kefir culture

PAGE 66

black tea for kombucha fermentation

kombucha SCOBY

PAGE 86

Jun SCOBY

PAGE 106

fresh unhomogenized cow's milk for milk kefir

kombucha SCOBY

PAGE 86

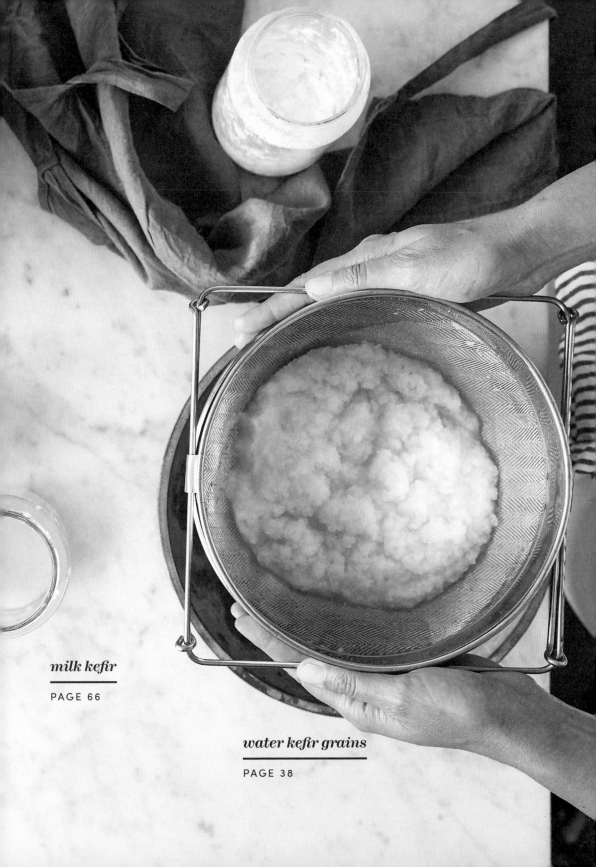

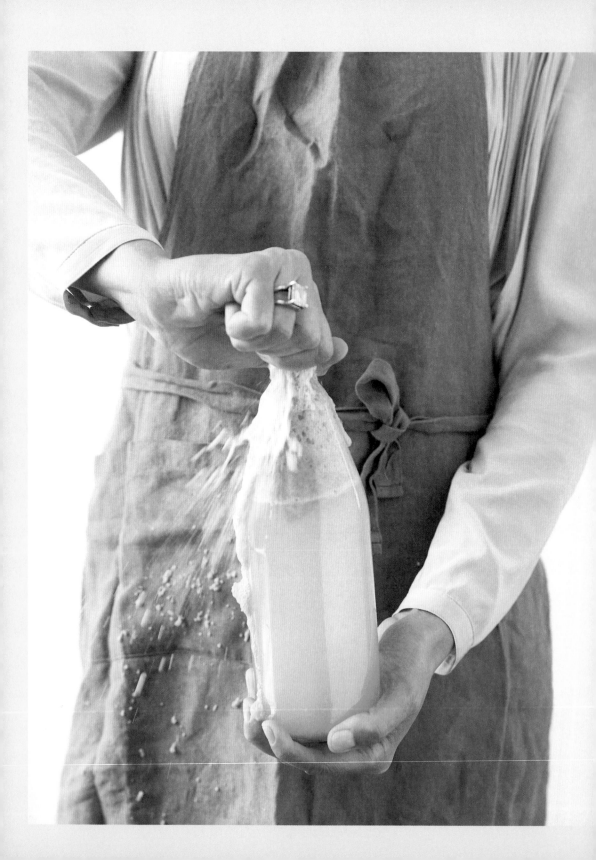

THE HOW AND WHY OF
FERMENTATION

In its simplest form, fermentation occurs when sugars are converted by yeasts and bacteria into carbon dioxide and trace amounts of alcohol, resulting in a low-sugar fizzy drink.

PRIMARY AND SECONDARY FERMENTATION

Generally, there are two stages of fermentation:
* **primary** (or first ferment)
* **secondary** (or second ferment).

Primary fermentation is the beginning stage where the ingredients are assembled and mixed together, cultures are added (if they are being used) and the fermentation starts. This period also encompasses the waiting time for the first fermentation to happen. It's everything that happens before you bottle the product.

Secondary fermentation is the period after the ferment is bottled and any cultures have been removed, and you are waiting for the carbonation to build and the flavors to develop. This happens in the bottle or jar, most of the time with the lid on.

HOW TEMPERATURE AFFECTS FERMENTATION

In my commercial brewery, I have invested in a temperature-controlled environment so that fermentation times are consistent, but this is not necessary at home. As a general rule, hot temperatures will speed up the primary and secondary fermentation stages, while cooler temperatures will slow down fermentation.

A range of temperatures is acceptable for home fermentation, but you will need to adjust the timings accordingly, allowing more time in cooler months and less time in hotter months.

Resting the cultures and storing the finished drinks in the fridge slows down fermentation. This means the taste remains balanced and the carbonation does not become excessive.

AEROBIC AND ANAEROBIC FERMENTATION

There are two types of fermentation covered in this book: aerobic fermentation and anaerobic fermentation. Aerobic fermentation refers to those ferments that require oxygen during the primary fermentation stage (e.g., Jun, kefir and kombucha). These ferments are covered with cheesecloth.

Anaerobic fermentation refers to those ferments that don't require oxygen (e.g., beet kvass, honey mead). These are covered with a lid during primary fermentation.

FIZZY FERMENTS

* Water kefir * Coconut water kefir
* Kombucha * Jun
* Pineapple tepache * Ginger beer
* Root beer * Honey mead

NOT-SO-FIZZY FERMENTS
* Milk kefir * Beet kvass

THE FIZZ

The fizz that develops in some ferments can be a sign of active fermentation and the transformation that has occurred, converting the sugars into carbon dioxide and a small amount of alcohol. As a general rule, the fizzier the finished product, the more alcohol it's likely to contain. Naturally fermented probiotic drinks can contain anywhere from 0.01 to 3 percent alcohol, with most containing around 1 percent. If you are concerned about the small amount of naturally occurring alcohol, you can dilute the drink using soda water.

Not all ferments produce strong fizz. Beet kvass and milk kefir, for example, are not fizzy drinks. It's simple: only the recipes that include added sugars, in the form of sweet fruits and sugar, will produce fizz. This does not mean that your finished product will be sugary. On the contrary, during fermentation the active yeasts consume the sugar, which leaves a low-sugar, fizzy drink. The sugar is for the culture, not for you.

Once bottled, the fizz will start off slow and gradually increase in force as the living yeasts and bacteria consume the sugars in the drink. They will peak at full force and you will have a decidedly fizzy brew. After the remaining

residual sugars have all been eaten by the yeasts and the food supply is gone, the fizz will reduce and the drink will turn vinegary and flat. It could take several months for this to happen.

FIZZ LEVELS OVER TIME

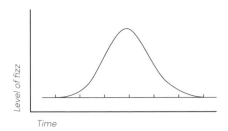

HOW TO OPEN A FIZZY FERMENT

Congratulations! You are holding a lovely fizzy bottle of probiotics in your hand. Here are three ways to open it so that you don't lose a precious drop.

* Open the lid slightly – but don't pull the cap right off – and allow the fizz to gush into a glass. Once the fizzy part is out of the bottle, you can take off the cap and pour as usual.
* Open the bottle in the kitchen sink, over a large bowl to catch the fizz. It can help to put a clean resealable plastic bag over the opening of the bottle so that the bag traps the fizz and it falls down into the bowl.
* Turn the bottle on its side and pour from that angle so that the fizz goes straight into your glass.

HEALTHY
FERMENTATION

Here are some broad guidelines to help ensure your ferments are the best they can possibly be.

Healthy ingredients = healthy ferments

Strive to source and select the best primary ingredients for your ferments. The quality of the produce you use will affect the end result. If organic ingredients are available, your ferments will be even healthier. Nonorganic dried fruits contain chemicals that affect the cultures, so definitely use organic dried fruits. I generally find that nonorganic sugar is fine to use if this is the only option you have.

Water

Use chemical-free water for best results. The chlorine, fluoride and other chemicals found in our modern water supply can kill the delicate yeasts and bacteria you are trying to cultivate. A readily available source of unchlorinated water is filtered tap water or spring water.

Salt

The only salts I recommend for fermentation are mineral-rich dry salts, such as Himalayan pink salt or unrefined sea salt. These contain high levels of naturally occurring minerals to feed the good bacteria and also create an environment that deters pathogenic bacteria. The additives used in iodized table salt can interfere with the fermentation process.

Temperature

Hotter ambient temperatures will speed up fermentation and cooler temperatures will slow it down, so adapt the time frames given in the recipes as necessary. In hot weather, you may need a shorter fermentation time; in cold weather, you may need much longer. As a guideline, room temperature is around 68°F (20°C), cool is below 68°F (20°C), and warm is around 77°F (25°C) and above.

Sunlight

Place your ferments out of direct sunlight, but not in total darkness. I have mine standing on the kitchen counter.

Fermentation vessel

A wide-mouth glass jar with a lid is all you will need for primary fermentation. You don't need to go out and buy anything special. Glass is best but you can also use food-grade plastic if necessary. As the volume of your ferments grows, you can gradually scale up to a 4-quart (4 liter) container that comes with a tap so you can pour the drink straight into your glass.

Covering

It is important to cover the fermentation vessel or resting cultures with cheesecloth, a loose-fitting lid or a loose-fitting plate where instructed. This prevents excessive carbonation from building up and causing an explosion.

Sourness and tartness

The finished ferment should taste tart and sour. Not only is this a sign of a healthy ferment, this sourness also stimulates good digestion so you can absorb more nutrients from your food.

Bottling

In general, using a bottle with a wide neck will give a lower amount of fizz and a bottle with a narrow, curved neck, such as a champagne bottle, will allow more fizz to develop. The shape of the bottle is important only when it comes to considering how bubbly you want your drink to be and making sure the bottle is sturdy enough to hold the pressure that builds as a result of the fermentation.

For most of the ferments I recommend using a narrow-neck bottle in the secondary fermentation stage so that you end up with a superfizzy drink. However, this is not essential. You can use any shape bottle you like or no bottle at all and enjoy the drink straight out of the fermentation vessel.

Cleanliness

I don't sterilize the equipment I use in home fermentation as the chemical residue can kill the good bacteria, plus it's an additional stage I have never felt necessary at home. Wash your equipment well in hot water with dishwashing liquid, then rinse it under hot water and leave it upside down to drain and air dry. Ensure your hands and utensils are very clean.

Labeling

I know you're going to get stuck right into the variety of ferments in this book and you might have several going at one time. Get yourself some masking tape and a permanent marker to name and date your creations.

Time is your friend

Patience is the key to fermentation: some things in life can't be hurried and fermentation is one of them. Fermentation is not an exact science and the results depend on a range of variables. Keeping a fermentation diary and recording notes about the behavior of each ferment can help you notice patterns and allow you to tweak your recipes as necessary. Carefully observing the fermentation process and developing your intuition is a large part of successful fermenting.

FERMENTATION TIME

There are a number of variables that affect how long the drinks take to ferment. As a result, the fermentation times given in the recipes are a guide only. These variables include:

* temperature
* the strength of the culture (where relevant)
* the quality of the ingredients used
* the type of water used.

Be patient and use your taste preferences as well as the fermentation guidelines and troubleshooting tips in the recipe chapters to guide you.

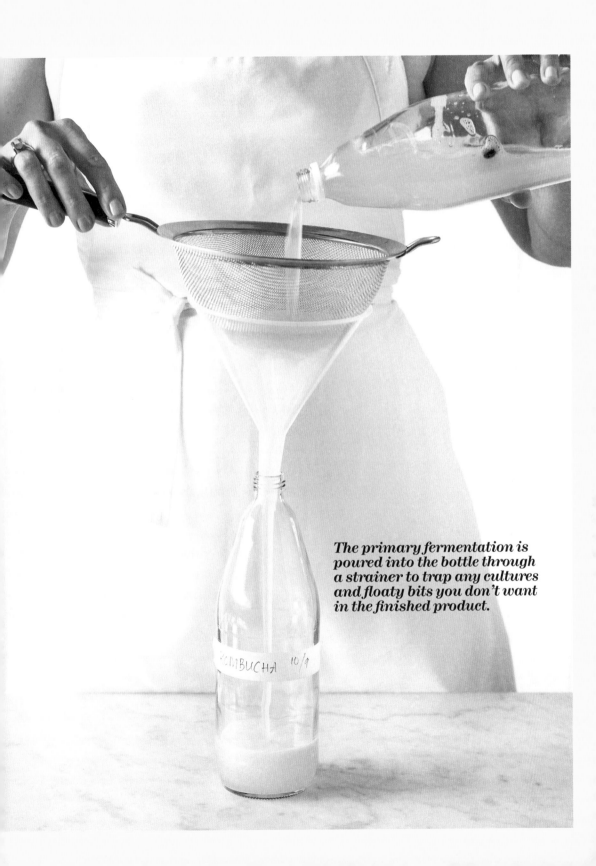

The primary fermentation is poured into the bottle through a strainer to trap any cultures and floaty bits you don't want in the finished product.

THE FERMENTATION
KITCHEN

All of the tools and equipment you need for fermentation are probably already in your home. Similarly, you probably already have the majority of the basic ingredients in your kitchen. If not, most supermarkets will carry these items. You don't need a lot of space to begin your fermentation journey. I recommend dedicating just a corner of your kitchen counter as a fermentation station. Remember to label each of your ferments with what it is and the date you made it.

TOOLS AND EQUIPMENT

Wide-mouth glass jars of varying sizes
Used as the vessel to ferment the drinks (I prefer glass jars but food-grade plastic jars are also fine)

Lids for the glass jars
Used to seal the jars for some ferments (e.g., beet kvass, honey mead)

Bottles of varying sizes with tight-fitting lids
To store the fermented drinks

Cheesecloth, dry dusting or other open-weave cloth, paper towel or unused coffee filter
To cover the vessel while fermentation is happening

Rubber bands
To secure the cover over the ferment

Funnel
To decant the liquid into a jar or bottle

Fine-mesh strainer
To trap the cultures or ingredients you don't want in the finished drink

Masking tape and permanent marker
To label your ferments with the name and date

Spatula/back of a spoon/wooden spoon
To push the milk kefir through the strainer, while retaining the intact milk kefir grains in the strainer

Immersion blender, blender or food processor
Helpful for pulverizing fruit and for making smoothies in the milk kefir chapter

Stockpot or large saucepan
For simmering the ginger and roots for ginger beer and root beer

BASIC INGREDIENTS

Filtered water
Either use bottled spring water, use a water filter pitcher or install a water filter so that you always have pure water on hand

Sea salt
Use pure sea salt, not iodized table salt

Honey
Buy the best raw honey you can afford to use for honey mead and Jun, and for sweetening the secondary ferment of your choice

Sugars
Have a supply of white, brown and raw sugars on hand for making your ferments – feel free to use a combination of sugars and see what you prefer (you can also experiment with other sugars, e.g., panela)

Organic dried fruit
The water kefir recipes need dates, figs and golden raisins

Molasses
Provides mineral content for the water kefir

Teas
If you have a basic tea selection, consider expanding your repertoire with a variety of teas that you can use in the kombucha recipes and for flavoring in the secondary fermentation stage for the other drinks

Coconut water
Either fresh coconuts or bottled coconut water will work

Herbs
Herbs can be found growing wild or in your garden, or purchased from the supermarket fresh or as dried leaves in neatly packaged tea bags

Roots
Ginger, galangal, turmeric and licorice are all fabulous roots to have on hand, either as a whole root, powder or in a tea bag

Spices and citrus zest
Star anise, cinnamon sticks, cardamom pods and orange zest are all fabulous for adding flavor to your drinks without adding sugar

Seasonal fruits
If there is a glut of seasonal fruits, freeze a portion to use later

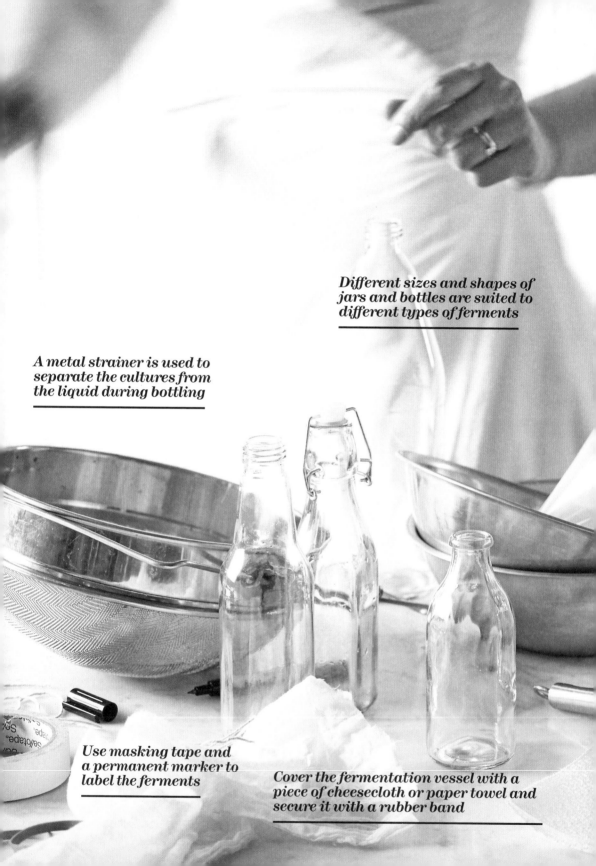

Different sizes and shapes of jars and bottles are suited to different types of ferments

A metal strainer is used to separate the cultures from the liquid during bottling

Use masking tape and a permanent marker to label the ferments

Cover the fermentation vessel with a piece of cheesecloth or paper towel and secure it with a rubber band

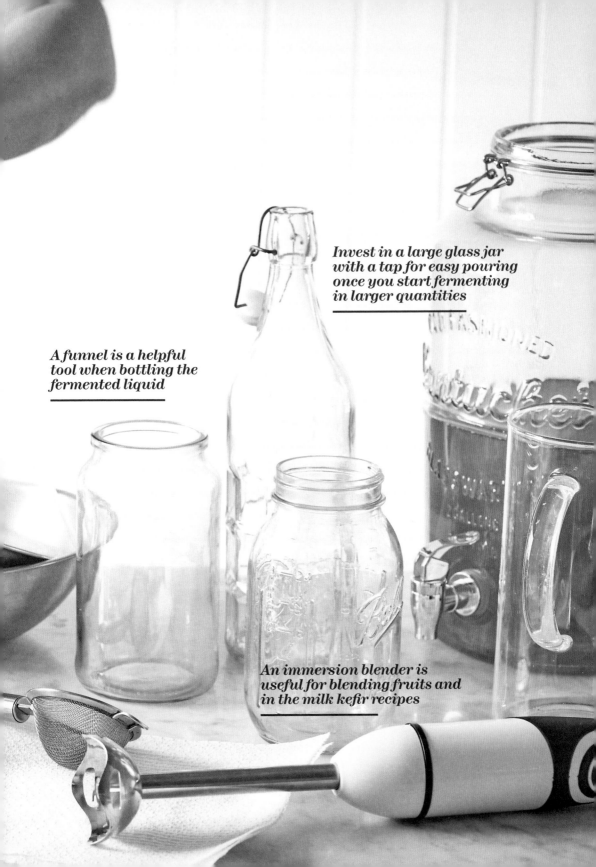

Invest in a large glass jar with a tap for easy pouring once you start fermenting in larger quantities

A funnel is a helpful tool when bottling the fermented liquid

An immersion blender is useful for blending fruits and in the milk kefir recipes

TO YOUR DRINKS

Boost the nutrient content of your probiotic drinks by including any of the following superfoods. Add them in the secondary fermentation stage, when the final drink is in the bottle and you are about to leave it to carbonate at room temperature. Most of these ingredients are available at your local drug, supermarket or health food store.

Chia seeds
Chia seeds are fabulous for boosting the omega-3 content of any of the drinks. They also add extra gut-healing goodness. Any color is fine: white, black or a combination.

Maca powder
Maca is a root that is grown in the mountains of Peru and is known to be an overall health booster. Add ¼ to ½ teaspoon of maca powder per quart (1 liter) as an extra dose of goodness in your finished drink.

Acai powder
The powdered form of the crimson acai berry, this superfood is packed with antioxidants.

Ginseng powder
Add an instant energy hit to any of the elixirs with Siberian ginseng.

Matcha
A powdered Japanese green tea, matcha has a herbaceous flavor and can add incredible antioxidant power to your drinks. Go easy, as a little goes a long way. Start by adding about ½ teaspoon per quart (1 liter) and build from there.

Chlorophyll
Chlorophyll is the green pigment found in plants. You can add powdered or liquid chlorophyll to any of your drinks for extra cleansing and alkalizing.

Fresh or dried cranberries
Used either whole or as a powder, these tart berries can add more flavor and increase the antioxidant profile of the final drink.

Spirulina powder
This superfood algae packs a lot of punch and is high in protein and antioxidants. Try adding ¼ teaspoon spirulina per quart (1 liter) of finished kombucha or water kefir.

Cacao powder/cacao nibs
Cacao is packed with antioxidants and that beautiful chocolate flavor we all love. Try adding a sprinkling to your water kefir or milk kefir milkshake.

Camu camu powder
Camu camu powder has an astringent taste and is loaded with vitamin C. Add a little to your drink for a vitamin C shot with your liquid probiotics.

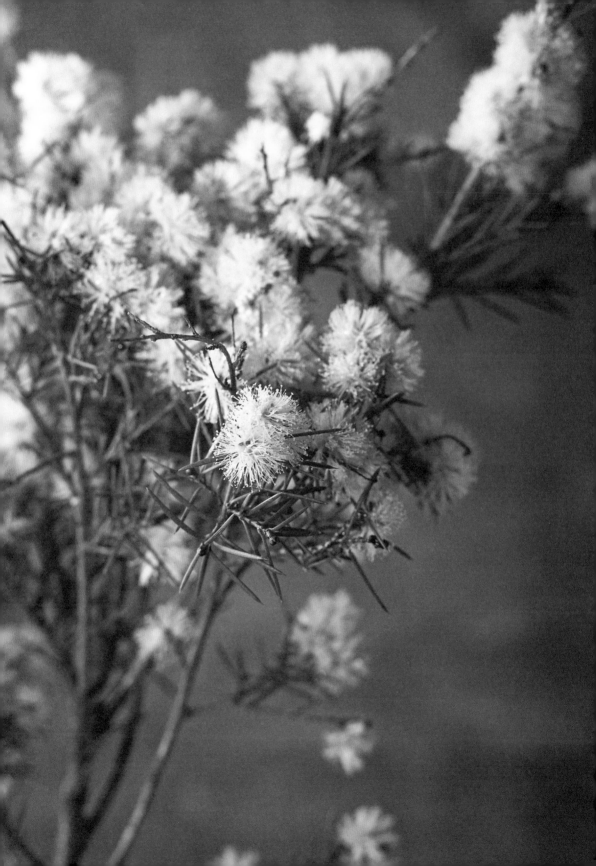

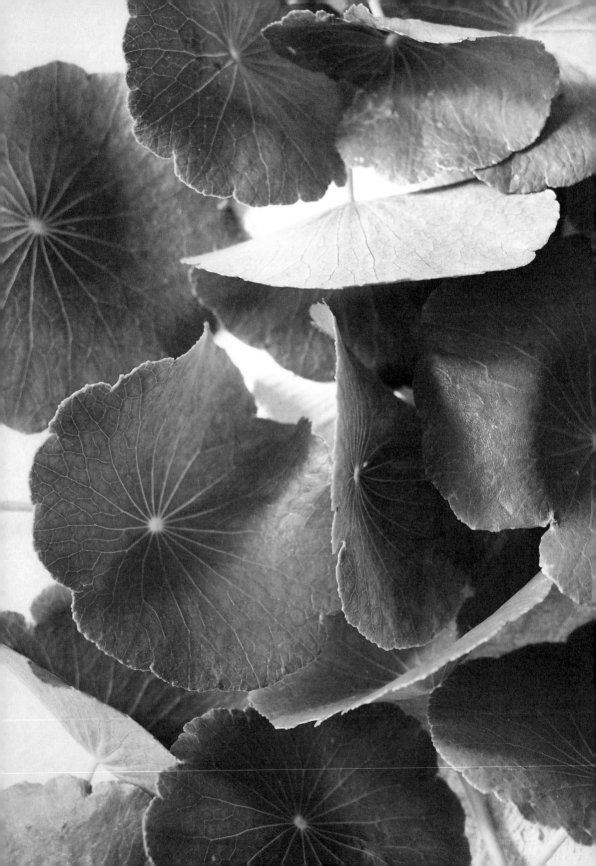

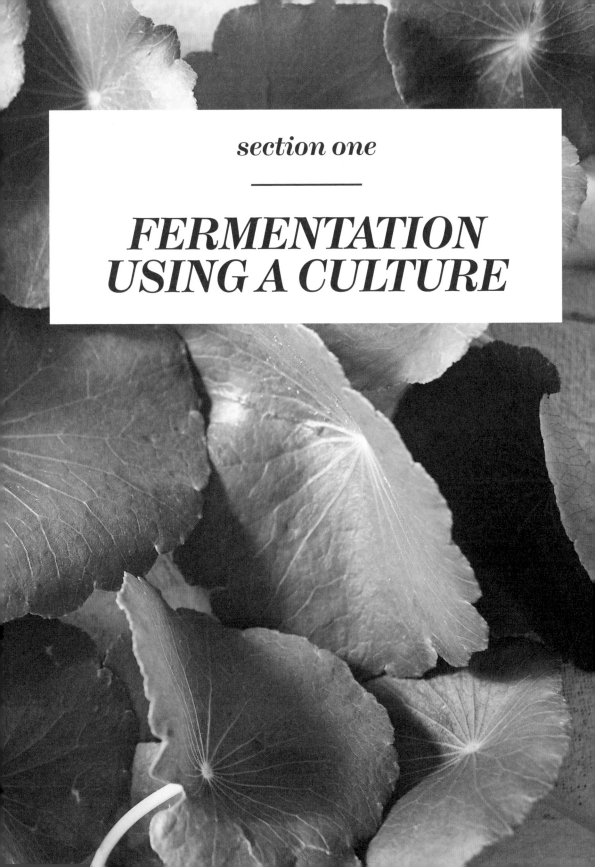

section one

———

FERMENTATION USING A CULTURE

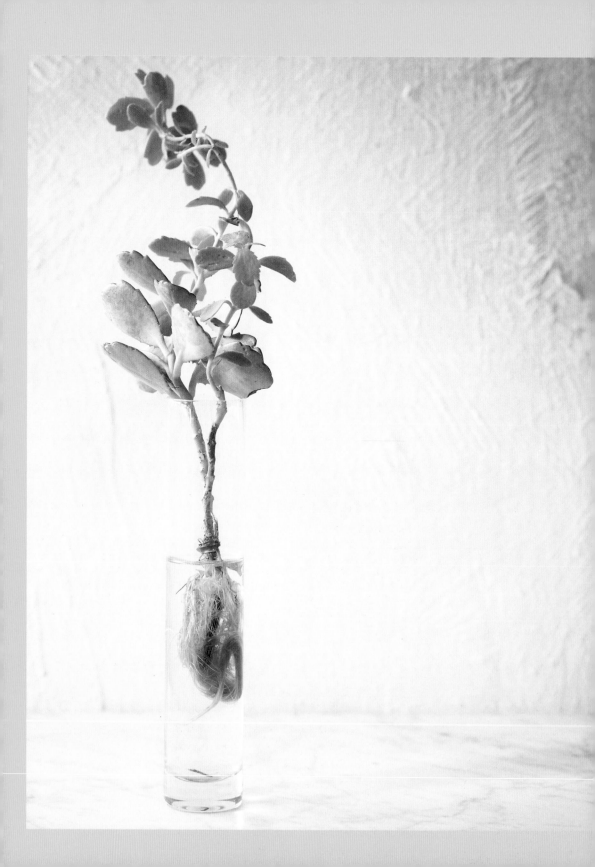

INTRODUCTION

Fermentation using a culture refers to any type of fermentation that requires a SCOBY (symbiotic colony of bacteria and yeasts) to seed the process of fermentation. The terms *Mother*, *culture* or *starter* are other names for a SCOBY, and these terms can be used interchangeably. For example, water kefir fermentation needs water kefir grains or water kefir culture to begin the fermentation, kombucha requires a mother or SCOBY, and sourdough needs a sourdough starter.

Each type of SCOBY is held together in a polysaccharide matrix – a web, if you like, to keep the collection of bacteria and yeasts together. Every SCOBY is unique to its location, environment and owners. For example, my kombucha SCOBY may look the same as yours but it could have a slightly different bacteria and yeast composition. They will both do the same job of fermenting sugared tea, but the finished products may be slightly different. These differences are an inherent part of the art and mystique of fermentation.

EXAMPLES OF FERMENTS REQUIRING A CULTURE

* Yogurt
* Milk kefir
* Water kefir
* Kombucha
* Jun
* Sourdough
* Skyr

All of the cultures have to be sourced from somewhere or someone. Some cultures are family treasures, passed on through bloodlines and kept as sacred heirlooms. These heirlooms could share a unique bacterial and yeast makeup specific to that family.

Think of these cultures as being part of your family, like a pet, that needs regular attention. Although they can generally tolerate some neglect they are reasonably delicate and will need regular feeding in order to thrive. Some cultures are hardier than others. For example, a kombucha SCOBY tends to cope better with neglect than water kefir grains. Refer to the guidelines and troubleshooting notes for each ferment type in the relevant chapter.

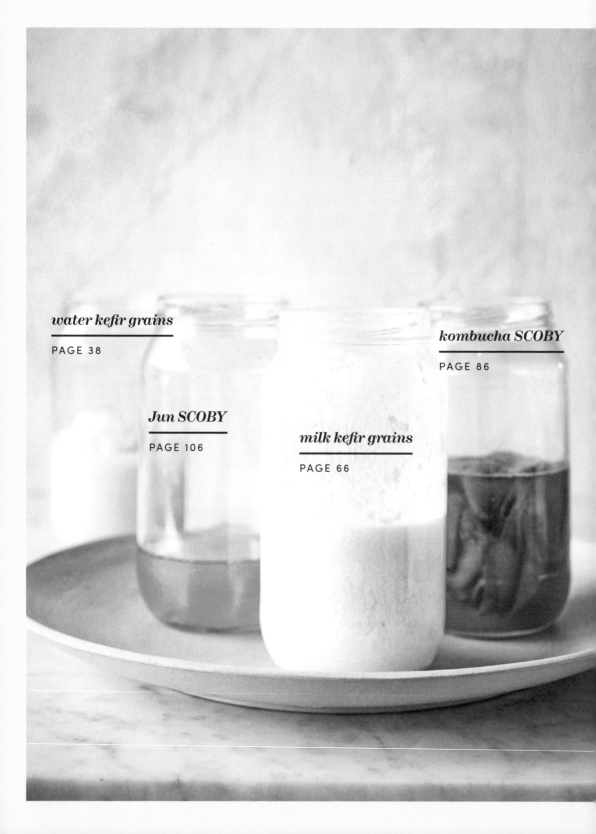

CULTURE
CARE

The cultures you use to make water kefir, milk kefir, kombucha and Jun can be kept indefinitely if they are cared for correctly. They can last a lifetime and continue to reproduce for generations.

In each recipe chapter, I have outlined the specific method of storing the culture if you need to stop fermenting for a time. Follow the guidelines and troubleshooting tips to ensure your cultures are active and healthy.

All healthy cultures will grow and reproduce over time. In general, water kefir and kombucha cultures multiply faster than milk kefir and Jun. With frequent fermentation, you could expect to see a doubling of the kombucha or water kefir culture about every 2 weeks. The growth is usually faster in the hotter months. Jun and milk kefir are generally a little slower to multiply, with Jun being particularly slow. With frequent fermentation, you can expect to see the culture doubling every 4 to 6 weeks or so.

Once your cultures have begun to grow and reproduce, you will need to reduce some of the excess culture. Otherwise, if the ratio of culture to liquid is out of balance, you may experience some of the following problems:

* there can be increased alcohol in the final fermented product
* the drink can ferment too quickly and turn acidic
* the drink can be syrupy
* the yeasts can take over, making the drink smelly
* the drink may not taste the way you hoped it would.

Don't panic! There is an art to fermenting, and you will develop a knack and get a feel for your cultures as you practice. There are plenty of fermentation guidelines and troubleshooting tips in this book to help you.

EXCESS CULTURE

Here are some ways you can deal with the excess culture.

Divide the culture and store the excess
Simply keep the amount of culture you need for the recipe and store the rest in the fridge, following the fermentation guidelines in the recipe chapters.

Give the culture away
What a lovely gift for someone! Package up the excess culture and give it to a friend with some instructions so they can start their own fermentation journey.

Increase the volume of water and other ingredients proportionately
If you want to make larger volumes of the drinks, just increase the ingredients proportionately as the culture grows. You may start making up to 5¼ quarts (5 liters) of kombucha at once with the excess culture.

Feed the culture to your chickens

Chickens tend to love the excess culture. Think of all the benefits your feathered friends will gain by eating the probiotics.

Compost the culture

If you add the excess culture to your compost it will speed up the decomposition process.

ROTATING CULTURES

Once you have excess cultures, I recommend you rotate the cultures that are in use with the excess cultures. This means the cultures have a rest from continuous fermentation. Follow the fermentation guidelines in each chapter to ensure they are stored correctly (in the fridge).

THE PURPOSE OF SUGAR SOLUTIONS IN CULTURE CARE

When you take a break from fermenting, the cultures can be stored in a concentrated sugar solution in the fridge. The solution serves as a concentrated food source for the cultures, keeping them well fed and nourished. Storing the cultures in the fridge, rather than at room temperature, slows down fermentation so that the cultures don't need to be constantly fed. When you are ready to start fermenting again, the cultures will still be alive because they have been stored in a wet, food-rich environment.

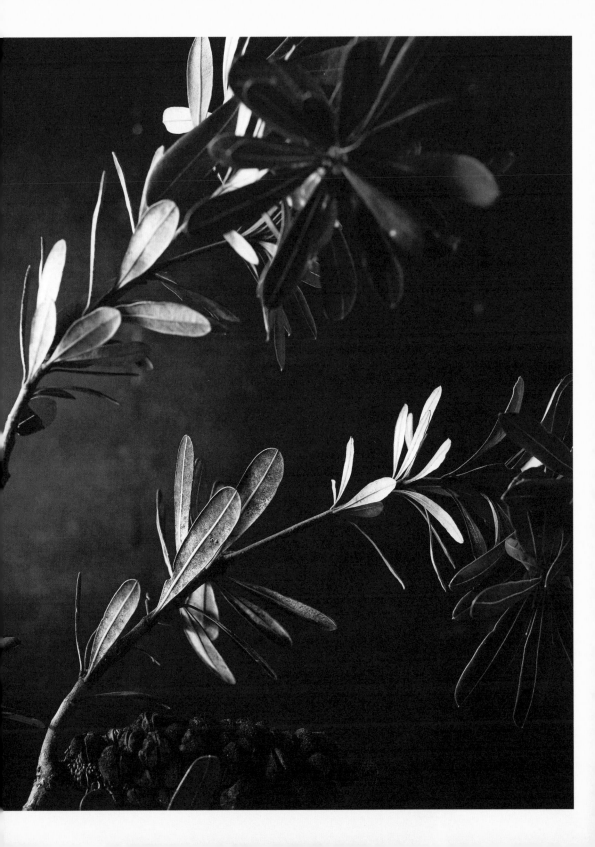

1. WATER KEFIR AND COCONUT WATER KEFIR

I drink water kefir every day and I'm convinced that my health depends on having this elixir in my life. It's my first love in the world of probiotic drinks and it's where my journey with fermentation began. Even though I have now made thousands of batches of water kefir commercially, it's still a thrill to watch the liquid transformation and hear the bubbling and fizzing that water kefir produces while it ferments.

WATER KEFIR CULTURE

Water kefir is known by many different names: water kefir grains, *tibi*, *tibicos*, Tibetan crystals, Japanese water crystals, SKG (sugar kefir grains), bees wine and California bees. The name "water kefir grains" comes from the grain-like shape of the culture, even though it doesn't contain any grains.

Water kefir grains are reported to appear on the fruit pads of the Mexican cactus, *Opuntia*. A report published in 1899 in the *Journal of the Royal Microscopical Society* explained that water kefir or tibi grains "ferment sugar-water and produce a light agreeable beverage."

Water kefir is a beautiful culture that appears as soft, jelly-like granules. These can be propagated effectively in a sugar-water solution. The culture looks like lots of clusters of translucent, gel-like florets that are shiny, bouncy and light, almost like wobbly jelly. It's a collection of bacteria and yeasts held together in a polysaccharide matrix – a web to keep the collection of yeasts and bacteria together.

Water kefir grains ferment a liquid that's rich in sugar and minerals, transforming the sugar into a probiotic-rich elixir. It contains different strains of living bacteria and yeasts. When you employ these bacteria and yeasts in a sugar-water factory, they will produce a beautifully refined, light and refreshing drink. Water kefir is easy on the belly and not acidic or strong like a kombucha.

The actual process of fermenting water kefir is simple. The tricky part can be handling the temperamental culture – water kefir needs a delicate balance of sugar water and minerals, as well as frequent care.

COCONUT WATER KEFIR

The water kefir grains love fermenting coconut water because of the high mineral and nutrient content naturally present in coconut water. Think of coconut water kefir as an adaptation of water kefir – instead of using a plain sugar-water base, it uses coconut water.

FERMENTATION GUIDELINES

Culture size

You need around ¼ cup (120 g) water kefir grains to ferment a 1-quart (1 liter) brew. When the culture gets bigger than that, you can increase the quantity of sugar water or coconut water proportionately or simply rest the extra culture in a sugar-water solution in the fridge (see page 40).

First fermentation vessel

Use a 6-cup (1.5 liter) wide-mouth glass jar or food-grade plastic jar to ferment the water kefir. Metal is no good for water kefir (you can use a metal strainer and utensils).

Covering

Water kefir is an aerobic fermentation process, so it likes oxygen in the first fermentation stage. Cover the fermentation vessel with a piece of cheesecloth or clean dry dusting cloth and secure it with a rubber band.

During the secondary fermentation, the bottle needs to be tightly sealed with a lid to allow the carbonation to develop.

Bottling

I recommend using a 1-quart (1 liter) sturdy glass bottle with a narrow neck and a tight-fitting lid. This allows the carbonation to develop and gives you a lovely refreshing, bubbly drink. You will also need a strainer and a funnel.

Position of water kefir grains during fermentation

Water kefir grains will generally sit at the bottom of the fermentation jar. Some clusters of culture will bob up and down during the active fermentation stage, looking almost like a lava lamp in movement.

Reusing or resting the culture

After bottling, you have two options for the water kefir grains. Either reuse the grains immediately in your next brew, or rest them in sugar-water solution in the fridge (see page 40).

Rinsing the culture

If the culture is looking stringy, has become smelly or seems otherwise uncharacteristic, briefly rinse it under filtered water. Otherwise, don't rinse the culture – just put it straight into fresh sugar water for resting or reculturing.

Taking a break from fermentation

The water kefir grains should be fine if they're immersed in sugar-water solution (see page 40) and covered with a loose-fitting lid or cheesecloth for up to 6 weeks in the fridge. It may take a couple of rounds of fermenting the grains in fresh sugar water to get the equilibrium back, so be patient.

RESTING THE CULTURE

If you want to take a break from making water kefir or have an excess of culture, you need to rest the water kefir grains that are not needed in a sugar-water solution in the fridge to slow down fermentation.

SUGAR-WATER SOLUTION

1 cup (220 g) raw sugar
1 cup (250 ml) hot water
3 cups (750 ml) filtered water or spring water,
*   at room temperature*
pinch of salt
1 tablespoon plus 1 teaspoon molasses
2 dried figs
2 dried dates

Put the sugar in a 6-cup (1.5 liter) glass or food-grade plastic container. Add the hot water and stir to dissolve the sugar.

Pour the cool filtered water into the container. Add the salt, molasses, figs and dates.

Add the water kefir grains to the sugar-water solution and cover the container with a piece of cheesecloth, a plate or a very loose-fitting lid. Store in the fridge for up to 6 weeks.

HOW TO KNOW WHEN YOUR
WATER KEFIR
IS READY FOR BOTTLING

SMELL
The water kefir should have a slightly sour smell – you will notice the change from sweet sugar water to sour and a little sharp. You should be able to smell a distinctive brewery or yeasty smell.

LOOK
You will notice the active fermentation happening – there should be lots of bubbles furiously peaking. It's amazing to watch!

LISTEN
There should be an audible, vigorous bubbling and fizzing sound as the water kefir ferments.

TASTE
The taste will change from sweet sugar water to tangy, a little sharp and a little sour. There should also be some bubbles on your tongue.

TROUBLESHOOTING

WHAT IF THE CULTURE ISN'T MULTIPLYING?

Healthy water kefir culture should reproduce over the course of fermentation. If you are brewing successfully but the culture is not reproducing, don't worry – the culture is a living entity and has times of rest and times of reproduction.

However, if the brew does not seem to be working and the culture is not multiplying, ask yourself the following questions:

Is your water chlorinated? All the ferments need unchlorinated water to thrive. Ensure you use a water filter or some other method like boiling the water to remove the chlorine.

Is your sugar too refined? Try using raw or light brown sugar and add a teaspoon of molasses.

Is the brew in the sun? Put it in a darker place.

Is it too cold or too hot? Water kefir prefers to ferment between 75°F (24°C) and 82°F (28°C).

Are there preservatives on your dried fruit? Make sure you use organic dried fruit as chemicals can kill the delicate balance of yeasts and bacteria.

WHAT IF THE CULTURE DISINTEGRATES AND BECOMES SANDY?

This could be due to a wide range of factors.

Sugar: are you using processed white sugar? If so, use raw or brown sugar.

Water: are you using activated carbon filtered water, tap water or demineralized water? If so, source mineral-rich water like spring water and see if that makes a difference. Don't use water that contains chlorine as this will kill the culture.

Minerals: are there too many minerals or not enough minerals? The recipes contain sufficient minerals for successful fermentation. However, every culture and water source is unique. Also, the mineral content of dried fruit can vary. This is why fermentation involves trusting your gut and using your senses.

Feeding times: water kefir needs to be fed every 48 hours during active fermentation, otherwise follow the guidelines on page 40 for resting the grains. If the water kefir has been fermenting for too long (longer than 3 days) and has consumed all the sugars, it could pickle itself in the acidic solution, starve and disintegrate. If this happens, it's probably time to source some fresh water kefir grains and start again.

WHAT IF THE CULTURE BECOMES MOLDY?

Occasionally (but unusually) mold can develop on your culture. Discard the culture and the water kefir and source a fresh culture.

WHAT IF THE WATER KEFIR IS OVERFERMENTED?

If your water kefir has a superstrong acidic smell and a musty taste, it may have over-fermented. Water kefir should be mildly sweet, pleasant to drink and taste beautifully light and refined. It should never be so strong that you don't want to drink it.

If the water kefir is overfermented, throw away the batch you just made and try again, making sure you don't allow it to ferment for too long, especially in hot weather. Only let it ferment for 2 days, or up to 3 days if you live in a cooler climate.

WHAT IF THE BREW LOOKS SLIMY?

How long are you brewing for? The brew could go slimy if it's overfermented. Only ferment it for 2 days, or up to 3 days in cooler climates. If you leave it for any longer than that it can become slimy. If this happens, rinse the water kefir grains and try fermenting them again following the recipe. It may take a few turns through the fermentation process to readjust and get the pH balance back.

The brew could also turn slimy if there are too many minerals. Try removing the molasses, salt and dried fruit for a couple of fermentation cycles and see if that fixes the problem.

RECIPES

basic water kefir

Although this is called "basic water kefir," in my mind there is nothing basic about it. Think about the complex arrangement and symbiosis between the water kefir grains, transforming a plain sugar-water mixture into a bubbling, living probiotic drink.

Preparation time: 15 minutes **Fermentation time:** 1½–5 days **Difficulty:** Medium
Shelf life: Refrigerate for up to 4 months **Makes:** About 1 quart (1 liter)

INGREDIENTS

¼ cup (55 g) raw sugar
¼ cup (60 ml) hot water
1 quart (1 liter) filtered water or
    spring water
pinch of sea salt
1 dried fig
1 dried date
10 golden raisins
¼ teaspoon molasses
¼ cup (120 g) water kefir grains

PRIMARY FERMENTATION

Put the sugar in a 6-cup (1.5 liter) wide-mouth glass jar. Add the hot water and stir to dissolve the sugar. Add the filtered water, sea salt, dried fruit and molasses and stir well to combine.

Add the water kefir grains to the jar. Cover the jar with a piece of cheesecloth and secure with a rubber band.

Place the jar out of direct sunlight at room temperature and leave the liquid to ferment for 1 to 3 days, depending on the temperature.

BOTTLING

Scoop out and discard the dried fruit from the liquid.

Put a funnel in the opening of a 1-quart (1 liter) glass bottle with a tight-fitting lid and put a strainer on top of the funnel. Pour the water kefir liquid into the bottle through the strainer. Set aside the water kefir grains in the strainer to reuse or rest (see page 40).

SECONDARY FERMENTATION

Tightly seal the bottle lid and leave the bottle in a warm place to build carbonation. This could take anywhere from 12 to 72 hours, depending on the temperature. "Burp" the water kefir daily to release some pressure by opening the lid slightly and then tightening it again.

DRINK UP

When the water kefir is as fizzy as you like (this could range from a small spritz to a ferocious fizz), store it in the fridge to slow the fermentation process, and enjoy cold.

lemon and ginger water kefir

———

This classic water kefir combination is dry, tangy and subtly sweet. The water kefir thrives on the raw ginger and you may see the culture replicating furiously, sometimes doubling in 24 hours. Don't squeeze the lemon juice into the jar at the primary fermentation stage, as it will tip the balance of acidity – just add the whole slice. In the bottling stage, you can squeeze the lemon juice into the bottle.

Preparation time: 15 minutes **Fermentation time:** 1½ – 5 days **Difficulty:** Medium
Shelf life: Refrigerate for up to 4 months **Makes:** About 1 quart (1 liter)

———

INGREDIENTS

1 recipe basic water kefir
   (page 44)
4 thick slices fresh ginger, skin on,
   cut into matchsticks
2 thick slices lemon
juice of ½ lemon

PRIMARY FERMENTATION

Follow the instructions for basic water kefir, adding half the ginger and 1 slice of lemon along with the dried fruit.

BOTTLING

Scoop out and discard the dried fruit, ginger and lemon from the liquid.

   Put a funnel in the opening of a 1-quart (1 liter) glass bottle with a tight-fitting lid and put a strainer on top of the funnel. Pour the water kefir liquid into the bottle through the strainer. Set aside the water kefir grains in the strainer to reuse or rest (see page 40).

   Add the lemon juice and the remaining lemon slice and ginger to the bottle.

SECONDARY FERMENTATION

Tightly seal the bottle lid and leave the bottle in a warm place to build carbonation. This could take anywhere from 12 to 72 hours, depending on the temperature. "Burp" the water kefir daily to release some pressure by opening the lid slightly and then tightening it again.

DRINK UP

When the water kefir is as fizzy as you like (this could range from a small spritz to a ferocious fizz), store it in the fridge to slow the fermentation process, and enjoy cold.

berry water kefir

Witness the beautiful berries imbuing the water kefir with their stunning color while they also infuse the liquid with their scent and antioxidants. If you're chopping the berries, make sure you eat them after their probiotic bath – they are full of goodness!

Preparation time: 15 minutes   **Fermentation time:** 1½–5 days   **Difficulty:** Medium
Shelf life: Refrigerate for up to 4 months   **Makes:** About 1 quart (1 liter)

INGREDIENTS

*1 recipe basic water kefir
     (page 44)
1 handful fresh mulberries,
     raspberries or other berries
     in season*

PRIMARY FERMENTATION
Follow the instructions for basic water kefir.

BOTTLING
Scoop out and discard the dried fruit from the liquid.

Put a funnel in the opening of a 1-quart (1 liter) glass bottle with a tight-fitting lid and put a strainer on top of the funnel. Pour the water kefir liquid into the bottle through the strainer. Set aside the water kefir grains in the strainer to reuse or rest (see page 40).

Purée or roughly chop the berries if desired and add them to the bottle.

SECONDARY FERMENTATION
Tightly seal the bottle lid and leave the bottle in a warm place to build carbonation. This could take anywhere from 12 to 72 hours, depending on the temperature. "Burp" the water kefir daily to release some pressure by opening the lid slightly and then tightening it again.

DRINK UP
When the water kefir is as fizzy as you like (this could range from a small spritz to a ferocious fizz), store it in the fridge to slow the fermentation process, and enjoy cold.

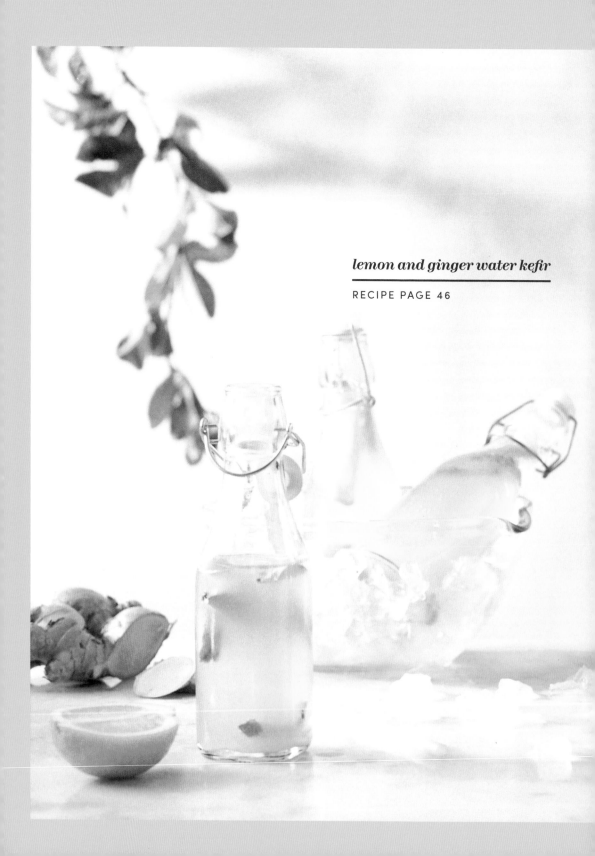

lemon and ginger water kefir

RECIPE PAGE 46

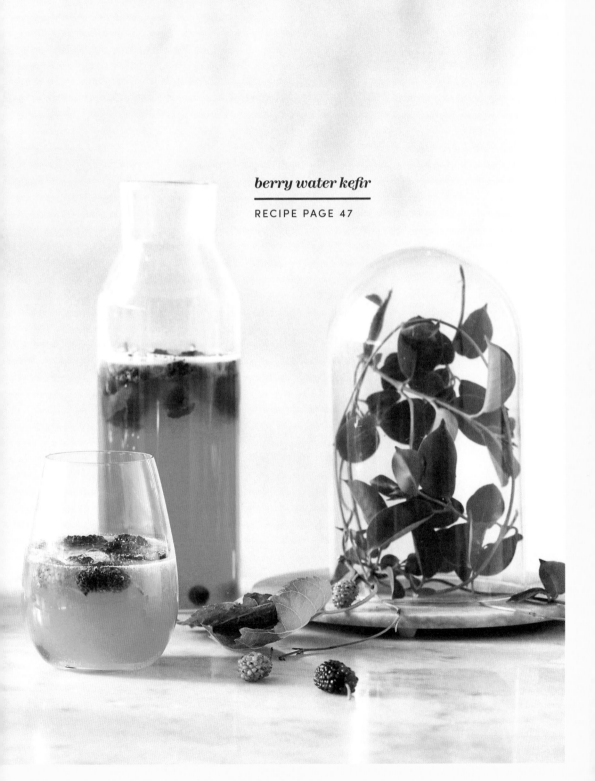

berry water kefir

RECIPE PAGE 47

pretty vanilla, rosewater and chia water kefir

The marriage of the delicate scent of rosewater with warming, creamy vanilla is very sensual and exotic. *Chia* is the Mayan word for strength and chia seeds are prized for their endurance and energy-giving properties. They are powerhouses of goodness, providing omega-3, fiber, antioxidants and protein.

Preparation time: 15 minutes **Fermentation time:** 1½–5 days **Difficulty:** Medium
Shelf life: Refrigerate for up to 4 months **Makes:** About 1 quart (1 liter)

INGREDIENTS

1 recipe basic water kefir
    (page 44)
¼ cup (60 ml) rosewater
1 tablespoon plus 1 teaspoon
    chia seeds
1 vanilla bean or ½ teaspoon
    natural vanilla extract
1 teaspoon edible dried rose
    petals (optional)

PRIMARY FERMENTATION

Follow the instructions for basic water kefir.

BOTTLING

Scoop out and discard the dried fruit from the liquid.

Put a funnel in the opening of a 1-quart (1 liter) glass bottle with a tight-fitting lid and put a strainer on top of the funnel. Pour the water kefir liquid into the bottle through the strainer. Set aside the water kefir grains in the strainer to reuse or rest (see page 40).

Add the rosewater, chia seeds, vanilla bean or vanilla extract and rose petals, if using, to the bottle.

SECONDARY FERMENTATION

Tightly seal the bottle lid and leave the bottle in a warm place to build carbonation. This could take anywhere from 12 to 72 hours, depending on the temperature. Give the bottle a shake every now and then to help disperse the chia seeds. "Burp" the water kefir daily to release some pressure by opening the lid slightly and then tightening it again.

DRINK UP

When the water kefir is as fizzy as you like (this could range from a small spritz to a ferocious fizz), store it in the fridge to slow the fermentation process, and enjoy cold.

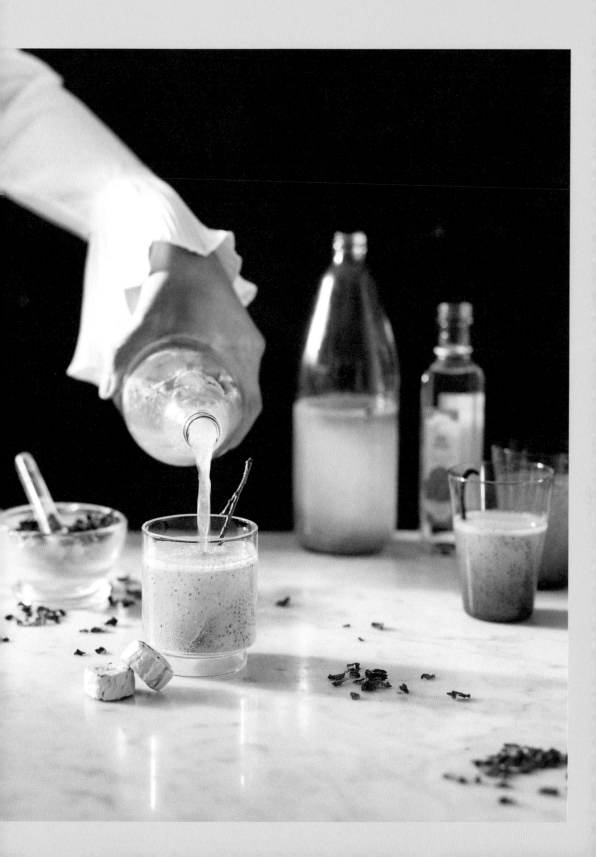

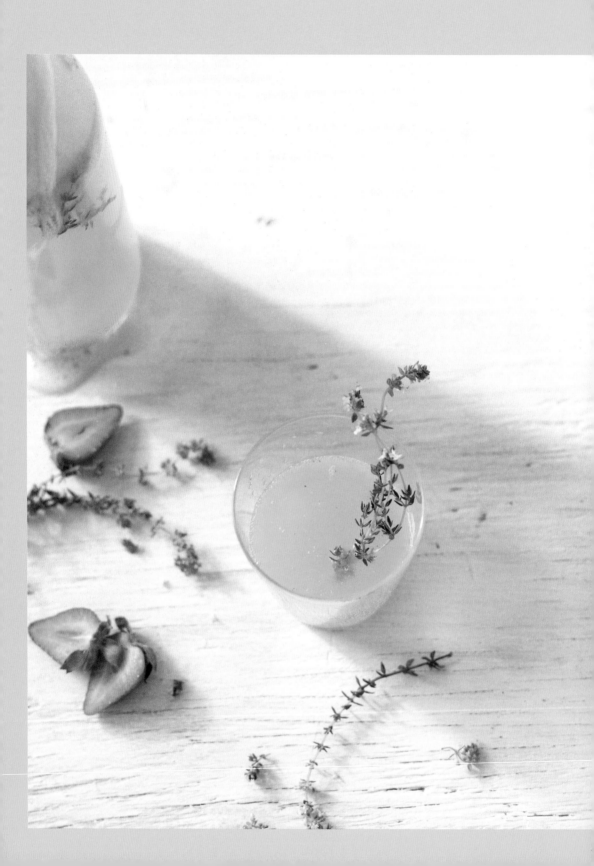

strawberry and thyme water kefir

The woody aroma and flavor of the thyme grounds the sweetness of the strawberries. This drink is simultaneously savory, sweet and tangy.

Preparation time: 15 minutes **Fermentation time:** 1½–5 days **Difficulty:** Medium
Shelf life: Refrigerate for up to 4 months **Makes:** About 1 quart (1 liter)

INGREDIENTS
*1 recipe basic water kefir
    (page 44)
1 handful fresh strawberries
3 thyme sprigs*

PRIMARY FERMENTATION
Follow the instructions for basic water kefir.

BOTTLING
Scoop out and discard the dried fruit from the liquid.

Put a funnel in the opening of a 1-quart (1 liter) glass bottle with a tight-fitting lid and put a strainer on top of the funnel. Pour the water kefir liquid into the bottle through the strainer. Set aside the water kefir grains in the strainer to reuse or rest (see page 40).

Purée or chop the strawberries and add them to the bottle with the thyme sprigs.

SECONDARY FERMENTATION
Tightly seal the bottle lid and leave the bottle in a warm place to build carbonation. This could take anywhere from 12 to 72 hours, depending on the temperature. "Burp" the water kefir daily to release some pressure by opening the lid slightly and then tightening it again.

DRINK UP
When the water kefir is as fizzy as you like (this could range from a small spritz to a ferocious fizz), store it in the fridge to slow the fermentation process, and enjoy cold.

Persian princess rosewater and saffron water kefir

Because water kefir has such a delicate and refined taste, the classic Middle Eastern flavors of rosewater and saffron really shine through in this digestive elixir. The beautiful color of the saffron creates a golden glow.

Preparation time: 15 minutes **Fermentation time:** 1½–5 days **Difficulty:** Medium
Shelf life: Refrigerate for up to 4 months **Makes:** About 1 quart (1 liter)

INGREDIENTS

1 recipe basic water kefir
(page 44)
3 saffron threads
¼ cup (60 ml) rosewater

PRIMARY FERMENTATION

Follow the instructions for basic water kefir.

BOTTLING

Scoop out and discard the dried fruit from the liquid.

Put a funnel in the opening of a 1-quart (1 liter) glass bottle with a tight-fitting lid and put a strainer on top of the funnel. Pour the water kefir liquid into the bottle through the strainer. Set aside the water kefir grains in the strainer to reuse or rest (see page 40).

Add the saffron threads and rosewater to the bottle.

SECONDARY FERMENTATION

Tightly seal the bottle lid and leave the bottle in a warm place to build carbonation. This could take anywhere from 12 to 72 hours, depending on the temperature. "Burp" the water kefir daily to release some pressure by opening the lid slightly and then tightening it again.

DRINK UP

When the water kefir is as fizzy as you like (this could range from a small spritz to a ferocious fizz), store it in the fridge to slow the fermentation process, and enjoy cold.

TIP *Serve the water kefir topped with cotton candy.*

summery watermelon and mint water kefir

The combination of watermelon and mint in this probiotic-rich water kefir makes a perfect drink for a hot day – it's fresh, cooling and hydrating. It's also a fantastic digestive aid. This is a living, fizzy, fruit soda drink that the whole family will enjoy, and lovely to take on a picnic.

Preparation time: 15 minutes **Fermentation time:** 1½–5 days **Difficulty:** Medium
Shelf life: Refrigerate for up to 4 months **Makes:** About 1 quart (1 liter)

INGREDIENTS
1 recipe basic water kefir
(page 44)
⅔ cup (100 g) diced watermelon,
puréed if desired
3 mint sprigs

PRIMARY FERMENTATION
Follow the instructions for basic water kefir.

BOTTLING
Scoop out and discard the dried fruit from the liquid.

Put a funnel in the opening of a 1-quart (1 liter) glass bottle with a tight-fitting lid and put a strainer on top of the funnel. Pour the water kefir liquid into the bottle through the strainer. Set aside the water kefir grains in the strainer to reuse or rest (see page 40).

Add the diced or puréed watermelon to the bottle with the mint sprigs.

SECONDARY FERMENTATION
Tightly seal the bottle lid and leave the bottle in a warm place to build carbonation. This could take anywhere from 12 to 72 hours, depending on the temperature. "Burp" the water kefir daily to release some pressure by opening the lid slightly and then tightening it again.

DRINK UP
When the water kefir is as fizzy as you like (this could range from a small spritz to a ferocious fizz), store it in the fridge to slow the fermentation process, and enjoy cold.

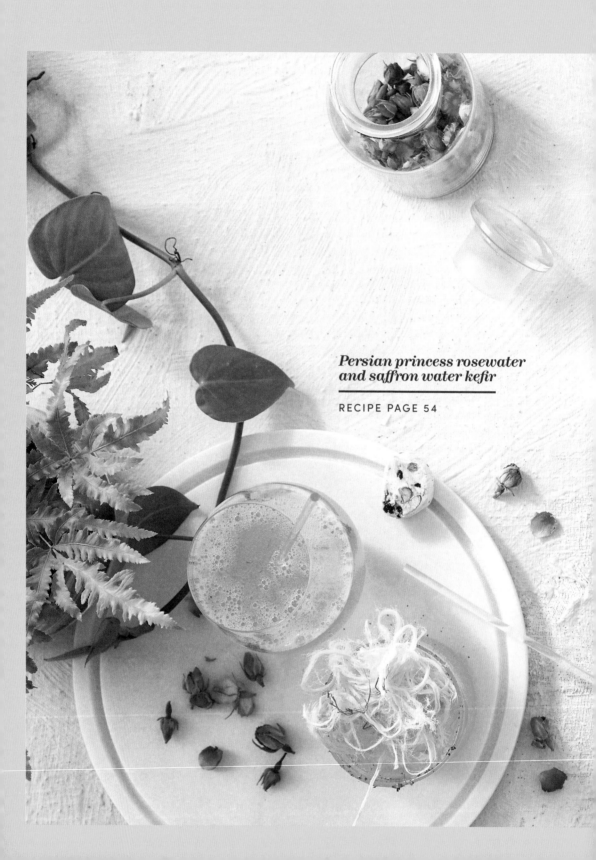

*Persian princess rosewater
and saffron water kefir*

RECIPE PAGE 54

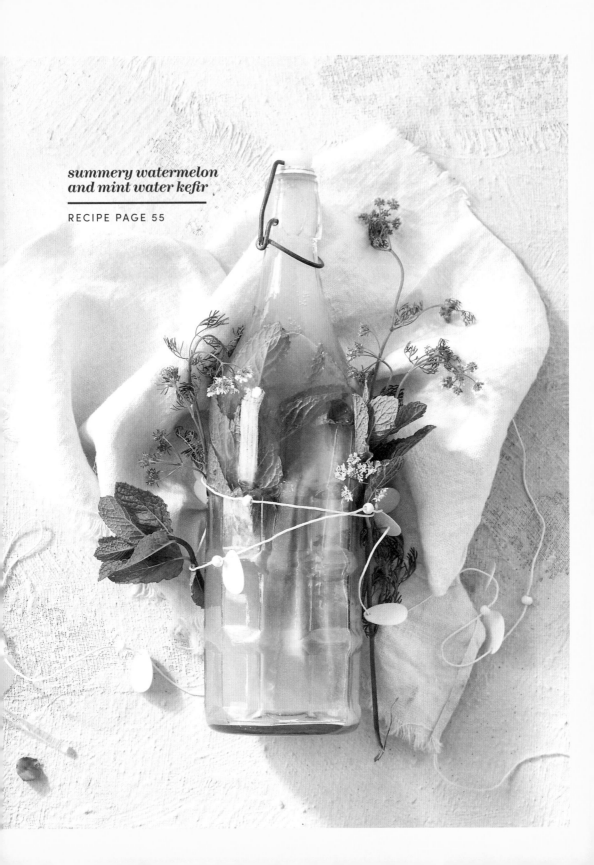

*summery watermelon
and mint water kefir*

RECIPE PAGE 55

RECIPES

basic coconut water kefir

Coconut water is a delicious way to ferment water kefir. It's naturally high in electrolytes and contains potassium, and water kefir grains love it – you may find they double their volume after being fermented in coconut water.
I use sugar in my coconut water kefir recipes because I find they work better with the added carbohydrate as food for the water kefir grains to ferment. However, if you are completely eliminating sugar from your diet, you can leave it out – just use the grains to make the basic water kefir (see page 44) after each batch of coconut water kefir so the grains don't starve. If you do leave the sugar out, please taste the brew after 12 to 24 hours, depending on the temperature, as the lower sugar content may mean
the coconut water kefir is ready sooner.

Preparation time: 15 minutes **Fermentation time:** 1–5 days **Difficulty:** Medium
Shelf life: Refrigerate for up to 4 months **Makes:** About 1 quart (1 liter)

INGREDIENTS

¼ cup (55 g) raw sugar
¼ cup (60 ml) hot water
1 quart (1 liter) coconut water
pinch of sea salt
1 dried fig
¼ cup (120 g) water kefir grains

PRIMARY FERMENTATION

Put the sugar in a 6-cup (1.5 liter) wide-mouth glass jar. Add the hot water and stir to dissolve the sugar. Add the coconut water, sea salt and dried fig and stir well to combine.

Add the water kefir grains to the jar. Cover the jar with a piece of cheesecloth and secure with a rubber band.

Place the jar out of direct sunlight at room temperature and leave the liquid to ferment for 12 to 48 hours, depending on the temperature.

BOTTLING

Scoop out and discard the dried fig from the liquid.

Put a funnel in the opening of a 1-quart (1 liter) glass bottle with a tight-fitting lid and put a strainer on top of the funnel. Pour the coconut water kefir liquid into the bottle through the strainer. Set aside the water kefir grains in the strainer to reuse or rest (see page 40).

SECONDARY FERMENTATION

Tightly seal the bottle lid and leave the bottle in a warm place to build carbonation. This could take anywhere from 12 to 72 hours, depending on the temperature. "Burp" the coconut water kefir daily to release some pressure by opening the lid slightly and then tightening it again.

DRINK UP

When the coconut water kefir is as fizzy and tart as you like (this could range from a small spritz to a ferocious fizz), store it in the fridge to slow the fermentation process, and enjoy cold.

healthy piña colada kefir

The classic flavors of piña colada immediately transport me to a world where coconut palms, a salty breeze and shootin' the breeze are de rigueur. In this virgin version, we welcome the health benefits of living probiotics, without the high sugar content and hangovers.

Preparation time: 15 minutes **Fermentation time:** 1–5 days **Difficulty:** Medium
Shelf life: Refrigerate for up to 4 months **Makes:** About 1 quart (1 liter)

INGREDIENTS

1 recipe basic coconut water kefir (page 58)

⅔ cup (100 g) diced pineapple, puréed if desired, or ½ cup (125 ml) pineapple juice

1 cherry or extra pineapple, to garnish each serving

PRIMARY FERMENTATION

Follow the instructions for basic coconut water kefir.

BOTTLING

Scoop out and discard the dried fig from the liquid.

Put a funnel in the opening of a 1-quart (1 liter) glass bottle with a tight-fitting lid and put a strainer on top of the funnel. Pour the coconut water kefir liquid into the bottle through the strainer. Set aside the water kefir grains in the strainer to reuse or rest (see page 40).

Add the diced pineapple, pineapple purée or pineapple juice to the bottle.

SECONDARY FERMENTATION

Tightly seal the bottle lid and leave the bottle in a warm place to build carbonation. This could take anywhere from 12 to 72 hours, depending on the temperature. This brew could create forceful carbonation. In order to prevent an explosion, "burp" the coconut water kefir daily to release some pressure by opening the lid slightly and then tightening it again.

DRINK UP

When the coconut water kefir is as fizzy and tart as you like (this could range from a small spritz to a ferocious fizz), store it in the fridge to slow the fermentation process. Enjoy cold, garnished with a cherry or pineapple piece for a tropical vacation feeling.

tutti-frutti coconut water kefir

This sensational fruity blend is best made with seasonal fruits that are at their peak – think nectarines, peaches, cherries, plums, figs, kiwi fruit and passionfruit. Add a handful to the coconut water kefir and watch as the gorgeous colors bleed into the white liquid and preserve that fruity summer flavor.

Preparation time: 15 minutes **Fermentation time:** 1–5 days **Difficulty:** Medium
Shelf life: Refrigerate for up to 4 months **Makes:** About 1 quart (1 liter)

INGREDIENTS
1 recipe basic coconut water kefir (page 58)
⅔ cup (100 g) diced seasonal fruit, puréed if desired

PRIMARY FERMENTATION
Follow the instructions for basic coconut water kefir.

BOTTLING
Scoop out and discard the dried fig from the liquid.

Put a funnel in the opening of a 1-quart (1 liter) glass bottle with a tight-fitting lid and put a strainer on top of the funnel. Pour the coconut water kefir liquid into the bottle through the strainer. Set aside the water kefir grains in the strainer to reuse or rest (see page 40).

Add the diced or puréed fruit to the bottle.

SECONDARY FERMENTATION
Tightly seal the bottle lid and leave the bottle in a warm place to build carbonation. This could take anywhere from 12 to 72 hours, depending on the temperature. "Burp" the coconut water kefir daily to release some pressure by opening the lid slightly and then tightening it again.

DRINK UP
When the coconut water kefir is as fizzy and tart as you like (this could range from a small spritz to a ferocious fizz), store it in the fridge to slow the fermentation process, and enjoy cold.

TIP *Frozen berries will also work well in this recipe.*

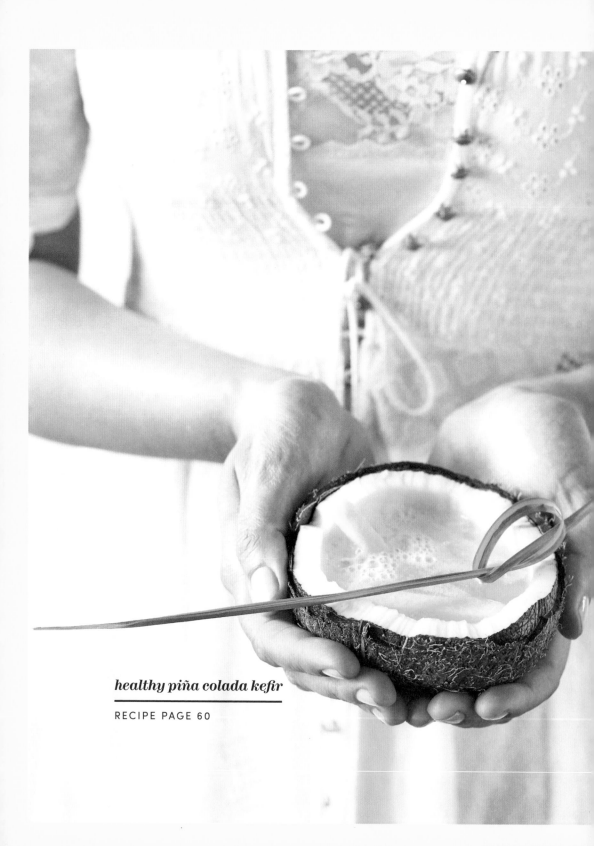

healthy piña colada kefir

RECIPE PAGE 60

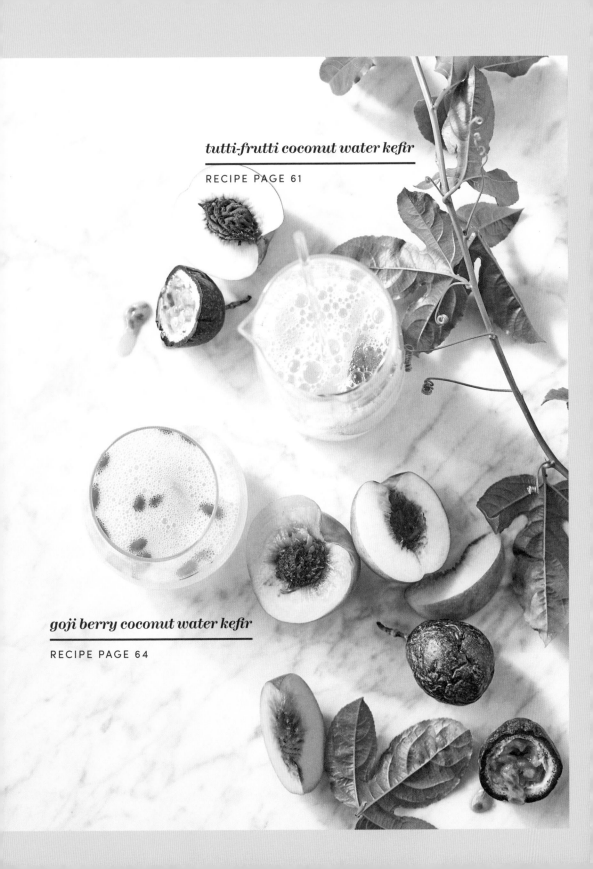

tutti-frutti coconut water kefir

RECIPE PAGE 61

goji berry coconut water kefir

RECIPE PAGE 64

goji berry coconut water kefir

Goji berries (*Lycium barbarum*) are one of the most nutritionally dense foods on earth. They contain all nine essential amino acids, a high concentration of protein, loads of iron, vitamin C, calcium, zinc and selenium, as well as powerful antioxidants to boost the immune system. Adding goji berries to a coconut water probiotic elixir, which is also rich in electrolytes, creates an incredible superfood drink. Make sure you eat the goji berries after their kefir bath.

Preparation time: 15 minutes **Fermentation time:** 1–5 days **Difficulty:** Medium
Shelf life: Refrigerate for up to 4 months **Makes:** About 1 quart (1 liter)

INGREDIENTS

1 recipe basic coconut water kefir (page 58)
1 handful dried goji berries, about ¼ cup (20 g)

PRIMARY FERMENTATION

Follow the instructions for basic coconut water kefir.

BOTTLING

Scoop out and discard the dried fig from the liquid.

Put a funnel in the opening of a 1-quart (1 liter) glass bottle with a tight-fitting lid and put a strainer on top of the funnel. Pour the coconut water kefir liquid into the bottle through the strainer. Set aside the water kefir grains in the strainer to reuse or rest (see page 40).

Add the dried goji berries to the bottle. They will swell in the liquid.

SECONDARY FERMENTATION

Tightly seal the bottle lid and leave the bottle in a warm place to build carbonation. This could take anywhere from 12 to 72 hours, depending on the temperature. "Burp" the coconut water kefir daily to release some pressure by opening the lid slightly and then tightening it again.

DRINK UP

When the coconut water kefir is as fizzy and tart as you like (this could range from a small spritz to a ferocious fizz), store it in the fridge to slow the fermentation process, and enjoy cold.

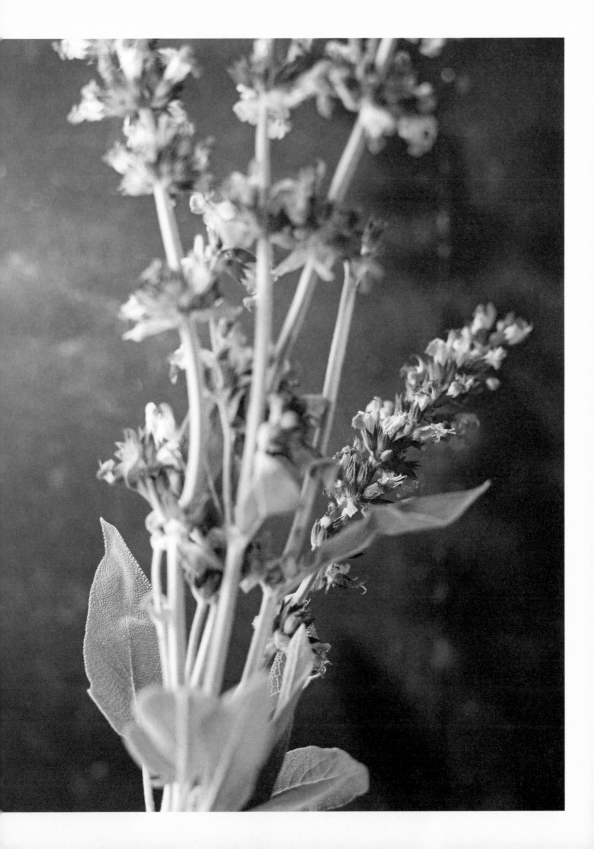

2. MILK KEFIR

Before the advent of electricity and fridges, milk from domesticated animals was soured in some form to preserve it, turning the milk from perishable to stable. Like all fermentation, milk fermentation is an ancient practice, with many cultures around the world having their own techniques and ingredients.

Milk kefir originated in the Caucasus Mountains. It was made and left to ferment in animal-skin bags hung near a doorway. Any time someone passed by the door, the bag would be knocked and thus the milk kefir would be kept well agitated. This agitation is an important part of the fermentation process, moving the milk kefir grains around the milk so they can get to the lactose to digest it.

During fermentation, the natural lactic acid bacteria in the milk kefir grains digest the lactose in the milk. Since the lactose levels in the milk are reduced, some people who can't digest milk find milk kefir an easily digestible product. The good bacteria responsible for souring the milk also protect it from invading pathogenic bacteria.

Milk kefir is also known as "milk champagne." When made correctly, it's a little effervescent and slightly alcoholic (generally ranging from 0.1 to 1 percent, which is normal for a fermented product). The taste and consistency can range from a little tart and runny to super thick and extremely sour.

Unlike yogurt, where some of the finished product can be used as a starter culture for the next batch, milk kefir must be made from milk kefir grains, which are also called a culture. You can't make this culture yourself – you have to acquire it from somewhere. The milk kefir culture is a cluster of bacteria and yeasts held together in a polysaccharide matrix. Like milk, it's white in color. It's a little slimy and bouncy to touch and looks like lots of small cauliflower florets joined together to form a cluster.

Given the right environment and nutrition, milk kefir culture can naturally self-reproduce and live forever. It will provide you with delicious probiotic-rich milk indefinitely, as long as you care for it. It's like having a pet in the house – it needs regular feeding and attention. Look after your culture and it will look after you.

THE STAGES OF
FERMENTATION

There are three distinct stages of milk kefir fermentation. Each stage produces a different type of milk kefir and each of these products can be used in a different way.

1. THICK MILK TEXTURE

This is the first stage and can be achieved in anywhere between 3 and 24 hours, depending on the temperature, the ratio of milk to culture, the quality of the milk and the strength of the culture. This stage is where the milk is inoculated with the milk kefir culture, but is not as far along the culturing journey as when it reaches a thick texture. It will be a little sweet and not as sour. It probably won't be effervescent, but it is still considered milk kefir. The consistency will resemble a thin, pourable yogurt.

2. YOGURT TEXTURE

This middle stage of milk kefir fermentation is generally reached between 12 and 24 hours. It's where the milk has been transformed into a thicker product, more like yogurt. This stage is perfect for smoothies.

3. THICK TEXTURE: SEPARATION TO CURDS AND WHEY

This is the fullness of the fermentation process where you will be able to see the separation of curds and whey. It generally takes the milk kefir between 24 and 48 hours to get to this texture. You will need to strain the milk kefir through a strainer to separate the curds from the whey. I recommend doing this overnight in the fridge in order to slow fermentation, using a bowl to catch the whey as it drips out. You can use the whey when making bread, soups, smoothies and stocks.

THE MILK KEFIR CURDS CAN BE USED IN A NUMBER OF WAYS

* Use them as a spreadable "cream cheese" on crackers or toast.
* Serve them as milk kefir soft cheese, with a sprinkling of sea salt, some chutney and crispy crackers for an afternoon snack.
* Spoon a dollop of the curds onto hot cereal.
* In bread making, add 1 tablespoon plus 1 teaspoon of the curds to the bread dough mixture to help with rising and fermentation.
* Add a spoonful to a smoothie.
* Cream the curds with honey and butter and use it as a spread on scones or toast.

MILK KEFIR
FERMENTATION GUIDELINES

Culture size
You need around 2 teaspoons milk kefir grains to ferment a 1-quart (1 liter) brew. When the culture gets any bigger than that, you can increase the quantity of milk proportionately or simply rest the extra culture in fresh milk in the fridge. A bigger culture will ferment much quicker and could also turn sour much quicker.

Milk
The higher quality milk you choose, the better quality the final product will be. Use a fresh whole organic unhomogenized variety if you can. You can also use goat's milk, sheep's milk, nut milk or coconut milk. If the culture is not fermenting the alternative milk efficiently, use cow's milk in the recipe for one or two batches of fermentation, then resume fermentation using the alternative milk.

First fermentation vessel
Use a 6-cup (1.5 liter) wide-mouth glass jar or food-grade plastic jar to ferment the milk kefir. Metal is no good for milk kefir (you can use a metal strainer and utensils).

Covering
Milk kefir is an aerobic fermentation process, so it likes oxygen in the first fermentation stage. Cover the fermentation vessel with a piece of cheesecloth or clean dry dusting cloth and secure it with a rubber band.

Bottling
I recommend using a 1-quart (1 liter) glass jar (like a pickle jar) or wide-mouth bottle with a tight-fitting lid for milk kefir. You also need a strainer and a 1-quart (1 liter) bowl that the strainer can sit over.

Position of milk kefir grains during fermentation
Milk kefir culture will float at the top of the milk. Stir the culture into the milk at least once a day to reincorporate it into the milk.

Agitating
Agitate the mixture as frequently as you can by stirring to reincorporate the culture into the milk. This could range from three times a day to not at all if you are away for the day.

Reusing or resting the culture
After bottling, you have two options for the milk kefir grains. Either reuse the grains immediately in your next brew, or rest them in fresh milk in the fridge (see below).

Rinsing the culture
If the culture is looking stringy, has become smelly or seems otherwise uncharacteristic, rinse it in milk. Otherwise, don't rinse it – just put it into fresh milk for resting or reculturing.

Taking a break from fermentation
The milk kefir grains should be fine if they're immersed in a 1-quart (1 liter) jar of fresh milk and covered with a loose-fitting lid or cheesecloth for 2 to 4 weeks in the fridge. It will take a few rounds of fermenting the grains in fresh milk to get them active and fermenting again, so be patient.

HOW TO KNOW WHEN YOUR
MILK KEFIR
IS READY FOR BOTTLING

SMELL
The milk kefir should have a slightly sour smell – you will notice the change from sweet milk to slightly sour.

LOOK
You will notice the active fermentation happening – the milk will thicken, it may separate and you will see clusters of milk fats and milk kefir culture in the milk mixture. You may notice a coagulation of thick milk kefir curds at the top of the mixture, sitting like a cork. It will look different at each of the three stages.

- **Thick milk texture:** it will still be liquid but thicker, like runny, pourable yogurt.
- **Yogurt texture:** it will be a standard yogurt texture, thicker than the "thick milk" but thinner than Greek yogurt.
- **Separation to curds and whey:** this is a distinct stage where there is clear whey at the bottom of the jar and thick curds that are the texture of cottage cheese at the top.

LISTEN
There won't be any audible sound of fermentation from milk kefir.

TASTE
The milk kefir will taste similar to plain unsweetened yogurt – tart, tangy, sharp and a little effervescent. The taste does not linger for long. Milk kefir does not have the thick viscosity and taste that fills your whole mouth that yogurt has; it's rather light, smooth and airy.

TROUBLESHOOTING

WHAT IF THE CULTURE ISN'T MULTIPLYING?

Milk kefir is a slower growing culture, so be patient – it will multiply in its own time. If you really want it to grow quickly, store it in fresh cow's milk at room temperature and keep refreshing the milk every 24 hours. You should see noticeable growth using this technique.

WHAT IF THE CULTURE DISINTEGRATES AND BECOMES SANDY?

The milk kefir culture should be soft, light and bouncy with the texture of set jelly. It's tricky to bring the culture back to buoyancy if it turns sandy and loses its jelly texture, so it's best to replace it with a fresh culture. There are many reasons that the culture could become sandy, including being fermented in milk that's not fresh and not rotating it in cow's milk if it has been fermenting in nut milk.

WHAT IF THE CULTURE BECOMES MOLDY?

Occasionally (but unusually) mold can develop on your culture. Discard the culture and the milk kefir and source a fresh culture.

WHAT IF THE MILK KEFIR IS OVERFERMENTED?

If the ambient temperature is hot, the milk kefir may only take 3 to 4 hours to ferment. In winter it could take as long as 3 to 4 days.

If your milk kefir has a superstrong smell, is very acidic and not palatable, it may have overfermented. Discard this brew, but retain the milk kefir culture for your next fermentation.

The brew may have overfermented due to any of the following reasons:
* the temperature was too hot
* it was left to ferment for too long
* there was too much milk kefir culture for the quantity of milk.

WHAT IF THE MILK KEFIR IS FERMENTING TOO QUICKLY?

To slow down the fermentation time, do one or all of the following:
* leave the mixture to ferment in a cooler place
* increase the ratio of milk to milk kefir culture
* increase the quantity of milk used.

WHAT IF THE MILK KEFIR IS FERMENTING TOO SLOWLY?

To speed up the fermentation time, do one or all of the following:
* leave the mixture to ferment in a warmer place
* increase the ratio of milk kefir culture to milk
* decrease the quantity of milk used.

WHAT IF THE MILK KEFIR SEPARATES WHILE IN THE FRIDGE?

This is normal and a sign of fermentation – just shake the bottle well before drinking.

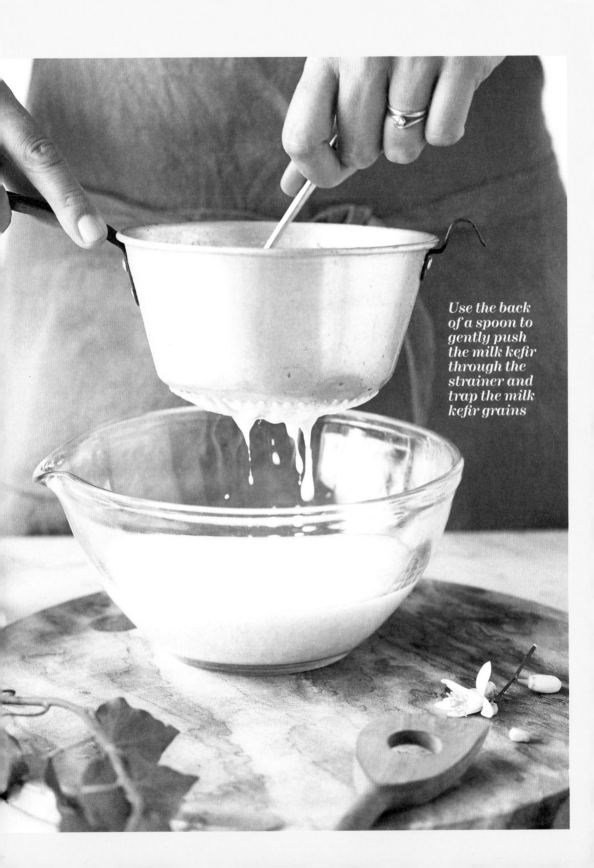

Use the back of a spoon to gently push the milk kefir through the strainer and trap the milk kefir grains

RECIPES

basic milk kefir

The finished milk kefir should be tangy, as well as a little zingy and tart. You may be able to feel some texture, which is the clusters of milk fats, yeasts and bacteria. It's perfectly normal for some separation to occur – this is the curds and whey becoming apparent. If this happens, simply shake the jar to mix it together. I choose to add cream to my milk kefir to make it thick and creamy, but it's completely optional.

Preparation time: 15 minutes **Fermentation time:** 3–72 hours **Difficulty:** Medium
Shelf life: Refrigerate for up to 5 days **Makes:** 1 quart (1 liter)

INGREDIENTS

1 quart (1 liter) whole milk
¼ cup (60 ml) whipping cream (optional)
2 teaspoons milk kefir grains

FERMENTATION

Pour the milk and cream, if using, into a saucepan. Gently warm, without boiling, to body temperature – around 98°F (36.5°C) or when you can comfortably leave your (clean!) finger in the milk for about 10 seconds.

Put the milk kefir grains in a 6-cup (1.5 liter) wide-mouth glass jar. Pour in the warm milk mixture and stir well. Cover the jar with a piece of cheesecloth and secure with a rubber band.

Place the jar in a warm spot out of direct sunlight and leave the liquid to ferment for 3 to 72 hours, depending on the temperature and the texture of milk kefir you prefer (see page 67). Agitate the mixture as frequently as you can to reincorporate the milk kefir grains into the milk.

BOTTLING

Set a strainer over a 1-quart (1 liter) bowl. Pour the milk kefir through the strainer so the liquid runs into the bowl and the thicker milk kefir is left in the strainer. Using a spatula, gently push the thicker milk kefir through the strainer into the bowl. The milk kefir grains will remain intact in the strainer. Set them aside to reuse or rest (see page 68).

Pour the milk kefir into a 1-quart (1 liter) glass jar or bottle with a tight-fitting lid and screw on the lid.

DRINK UP

Store the milk kefir in the fridge and enjoy cold.

honey and vanilla ambrosia

In Greek mythology, ambrosia is the food of the gods, giving immortality to anyone who drinks it. The combination of honey and vanilla is one of life's great pleasures. It's rich, warming, inviting and absolutely divine.

You can make the basic milk kefir ahead of time and store it in the fridge until you're ready to add the honey and vanilla. Alternatively, you can make the ambrosia and store it in the fridge for up to 5 days.

Preparation time: 15 minutes **Fermentation time:** 3–72 hours **Difficulty:** Medium
Shelf life: Refrigerate for up to 5 days **Makes:** About 1 quart (1 liter)

INGREDIENTS
1 recipe basic milk kefir (page 72)
*1 tablespoon plus 1 teaspoon raw
   honey*
1 teaspoon natural vanilla extract

FERMENTATION
Follow the instructions for basic milk kefir.

BOTTLING
Follow the straining instructions for basic milk kefir.
   Pour the milk kefir into a 1-quart (1 liter) glass jar or bottle with a tight-fitting lid. Add the honey and vanilla and either blend with an immersion blender, if using a jar, or screw on the jar or bottle lid and shake vigorously to incorporate well.

DRINK UP
Pour the ambrosia into glasses and serve immediately. Alternatively, store in the fridge and enjoy cold.

TIP *You can use this recipe as a face mask. Apply it to your face for up to 20 minutes for a natural skin conditioning treatment.*

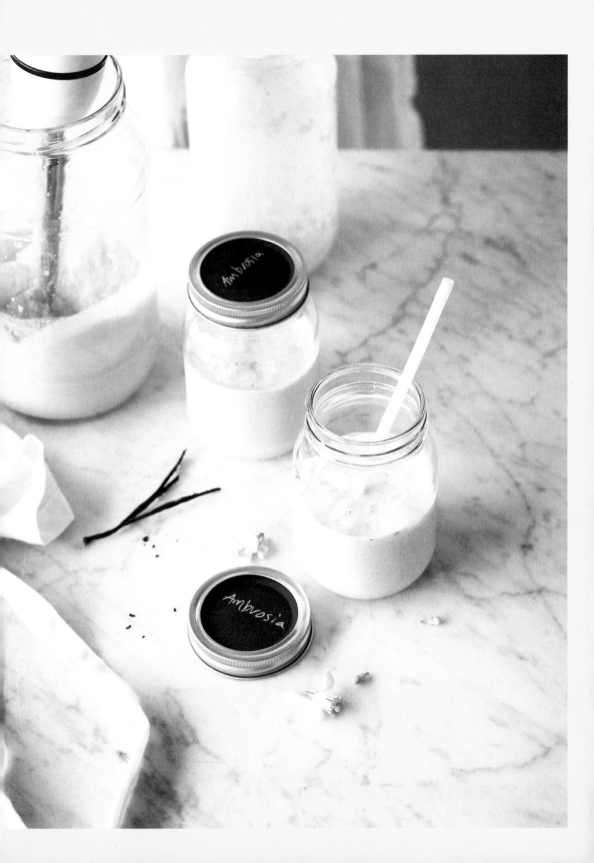

apple crumble shake

Warming, comforting and ultra nutritious, this shake is perfect at any time of the day – for a quick breakfast to tote to work, a dessert or an afternoon snack. I like to use the whole apple – skin, core and all – to increase the fiber and prebiotic content. The crunchy granola topping gives it more sustenance and texture, and adds extra fiber for healthy digestion.

You can make the milk kefir ahead of time and store it in the fridge until you're ready to serve the shake. Alternatively, you can make the shake and store it in a glass jar or bottle for up to 2 days in the fridge. Give it a shake and add the crunchy granola just before you serve it.

Preparation time: 15 minutes   **Fermentation time:** 3–72 hours   **Difficulty:** Medium
Shelf life: Refrigerate for up to 2 days   **Makes:** About 6 cups (1.5 liters)

INGREDIENTS

1 recipe basic milk kefir (page 72)
1 apple, quartered
1 tablespoon plus 1 teaspoon raw honey
1 teaspoon ground cinnamon
1 handful crunchy granola or muesli, to serve

FERMENTATION
Follow the instructions for basic milk kefir.

BOTTLING
Follow the straining instructions for basic milk kefir.

Add the apple quarters, honey and cinnamon to a high-speed blender and pulverize so that the apple is finely chopped. Pour in the milk kefir and blend until well combined. Alternatively, simply grate the apple and then blend it with the honey, cinnamon and milk kefir in a jar.

DRINK UP
Pour the milkshake into glasses and serve immediately, sprinkled with the granola or muesli. Alternatively, pour the milkshake into a 6-cup (1.5 liter) glass jar or bottle with a tight-fitting lid, store in the fridge and enjoy cold.

chocolate, cashew and chia shake

This shake is a taste sensation. In addition to the benefits of the living probiotics in every glass of milk kefir, it delivers antioxidants from the cacao, the gut-loving and soothing prebiotics of chia seeds and good fat and protein in the cashew nuts.

You can make the milk kefir ahead of time and store it in the fridge until you're ready to serve the shake. Alternatively, you can make the shake and store it in a glass jar or bottle for up to 2 days in the fridge. Give it a shake before you serve it.

Preparation time: 15 minutes **Fermentation time:** 3–72 hours **Difficulty:** Medium
Shelf life: Refrigerate for up to 2 days **Makes:** About 1 quart (1 liter)

INGREDIENTS

1 recipe basic milk kefir (page 72)
2 tablespoons plus 2 teaspoons
    raw cacao powder, or to taste
2 tablespoons plus 2 teaspoons
    hydrated chia seeds (see Tips)
1 handful raw cashew nuts
1 tablespoon plus 1 teaspoon raw
    honey (optional)
raw cacao nibs (optional),
    to serve

FERMENTATION
Follow the instructions for basic milk kefir.

BOTTLING
Follow the straining instructions for basic milk kefir.
    Add the cacao powder, hydrated chia seeds, cashews and honey, if using, to a high-speed blender. Pour in the milk kefir and blend until well combined.

DRINK UP
Pour the milkshake into glasses and serve immediately, sprinkled with raw cacao nibs, if using. Alternatively, pour the milkshake into a 1-quart (1 liter) glass jar or bottle with a tight-fitting lid, store in the fridge and enjoy cold.

TIPS *To hydrate the chia seeds, put them in a container, cover with cold water and then set aside for 10 to 20 minutes or until they plump up and swell to double their size.*
    Use any raw unsalted nuts you have on hand to make this shake.
    Serve the shake topped with cotton candy.

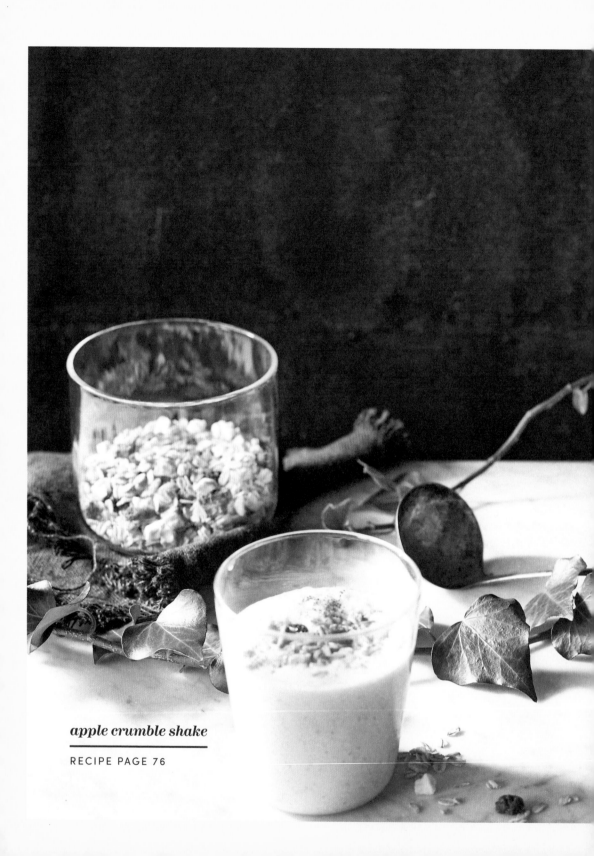

apple crumble shake

RECIPE PAGE 76

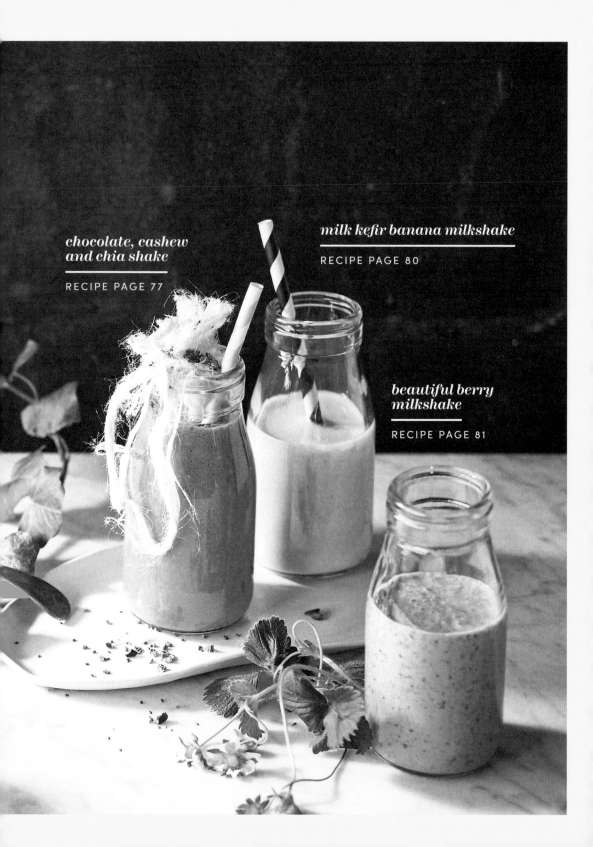

chocolate, cashew and chia shake

RECIPE PAGE 77

milk kefir banana milkshake

RECIPE PAGE 80

beautiful berry milkshake

RECIPE PAGE 81

milk kefir banana milkshake

_____

This probiotic-rich, belly-loving milkshake will have the kids lining up for more. I give this to my children every morning and they love it. Bananas are a good source of vitamin B6, manganese, vitamin C, potassium and dietary fiber.

You can make the milk kefir ahead of time and store it in the fridge until you're ready to add the banana and honey and serve the shake. Alternatively, you can make the shake and store it in a glass jar or bottle for up to 2 days in the fridge. Give it a shake before you serve it.

Preparation time: 15 minutes **Fermentation time:** 3–72 hours **Difficulty:** Medium
Shelf life: Refrigerate for up to 2 days **Makes:** About 6 cups (1.5 liters)

_____

INGREDIENTS

1 recipe basic milk kefir (page 72)
2 fresh or frozen bananas
1 tablespoon plus 1 teaspoon raw honey (optional)
ground cinnamon or freshly grated nutmeg, to serve (optional)

FERMENTATION
Follow the instructions for basic milk kefir.

BOTTLING
Follow the straining instructions for basic milk kefir.

Add the bananas and honey, if using, to a high-speed blender. Pour in the milk kefir and blend until well combined.

DRINK UP
Pour the milkshake into glasses and serve immediately, sprinkled with cinnamon or nutmeg, if using. Alternatively, pour the milkshake into a 6-cup (1.5 liter) glass jar or bottle with a tight-fitting lid, store in the fridge and enjoy cold.

___

VARIATION _To increase the protein content and give the milkshake a creamier texture, add a handful of ice cubes and 2 egg whites at the blending stage. This variation is best consumed immediately._

___

beautiful berry milkshake

Berries are high on my list of superfoods. Packed with antioxidants, including anthocyanins, quercetin and vitamin C, they fight oxidative stress that's caused by free radical damage. Plus, they are a taste sensation. This kid-friendly milkshake is nutrient-dense and it's packed with good bacteria to encourage excellent gut health.

You can make the milk kefir ahead of time and store it in the fridge until you're ready to serve the shake. Alternatively, you can make the shake and store it in a glass jar or bottle for up to 2 days in the fridge. Give it a shake before you serve it.

Preparation time: 15 minutes **Fermentation time:** 3–72 hours **Difficulty:** Medium
Shelf life: Refrigerate for up to 2 days **Makes:** About 6 cups (1.5 liters)

INGREDIENTS
1 recipe basic milk kefir (page 72)
1 cup (125 g) frozen berries
*2 tablespoons plus 2 teaspoons
    raw honey (optional)*
*goji or other berries (optional),
    to serve*

FERMENTATION
Follow the instructions for basic milk kefir.

BOTTLING
Follow the straining instructions for basic milk kefir.

Add the frozen berries and honey, if using, to a high-speed blender. Pour in the milk kefir and blend until well combined.

DRINK UP
Pour the milkshake into glasses and serve immediately, topped with goji or other berries, if using. Alternatively, pour the milkshake into a 6-cup (1.5 liter) glass jar or bottle with a tight-fitting lid, store in the fridge and enjoy cold.

TIP *Add a handful of ice if you want a supercold shake.*

---

sugar and cinnamon spice shake

The warming spices in this recipe work in harmony with the living probiotics to improve digestion and warm the body. Adapt the chai-style spice blend to include your favourite spices.

You can make the milk kefir ahead of time and store it in the fridge until you're ready to serve the shake. Alternatively, you can make the shake and store it in a glass jar or bottle for up to 2 days in the fridge. Give it a shake before you serve it.

Preparation time: 15 minutes **Fermentation time:** 3–72 hours **Difficulty:** Medium
Shelf life: Refrigerate for up to 2 days **Makes:** About 1 quart (1 liter)

INGREDIENTS
1 recipe basic milk kefir (page 72)
2 teaspoons spice blend (below)
2 tablespoons plus 2 teaspoons
    panela sugar
ground cinnamon and
    cardamom pods, to serve

SPICE BLEND
1 teaspoon ground cinnamon
¾-inch (2 cm) piece fresh
    ginger, skin on, or
    2 teaspoons ground ginger
2 cloves
pinch of ground black pepper
1 teaspoon fennel seeds
5 cardamom pods

Grind the spices in a mortar and pestle or spice grinder. Store in an airtight container in the fridge for a few weeks.

FERMENTATION
Follow the instructions for basic milk kefir.

BOTTLING
Follow the straining instructions for basic milk kefir.

Pour the milk kefir into a high-speed blender. Add the spice blend and sugar and blend until well combined. Alternatively, blend the milk kefir with the spice blend and sugar in a jar.

DRINK UP
Pour the milkshake into glasses and serve immediately, sprinkled with ground cinnamon and cardamom pods. Alternatively, pour the milkshake into a 1-quart (1 liter) glass jar or bottle with a tight-fitting lid, store in the fridge and enjoy cold.

TIP *You can also use the spice blend to make a milky chai drink. Infuse the spice blend in hot milk, strain and enjoy.*

Persian mint drink

I recently went to a beautiful Persian restaurant and as a welcome drink I was served *doogh*, which is a traditional savory yogurt-based digestive. The word *doogh* derives from the Persian *dooshidan*, meaning milking. Think of the classic Indian mango lassi as a sweet cousin of this savory version. Instead of yogurt, which is traditionally used to make doogh, I've used milk kefir in this version. It's just as delicious and packs a probiotic punch.

You can make the milk kefir ahead of time and store it in the fridge until you're ready to serve the drink. Alternatively, you can make the drink and store it in a glass jar or bottle for up to 2 days in the fridge. Give it a shake before you serve it.

Preparation time: 15 minutes **Fermentation time:** 3–72 hours **Difficulty:** Medium
Shelf life: Refrigerate for up to 2 days **Makes:** About 6 cups (1.5 liters)

INGREDIENTS

1 recipe basic milk kefir (page 72)
1 handful fresh or dried mint
    leaves
¼ teaspoon sea salt
2 cups (500 ml) sparkling or still
    water
cotton candy and edible dried
    rose petals (optional), to serve

FERMENTATION
Follow the instructions for basic milk kefir.

BOTTLING
Follow the straining instructions for basic milk kefir.

Pour the milk kefir into a high-speed blender. Add the mint leaves and sea salt and blend until well combined. Alternatively, blend the milk kefir with the mint and salt in a jar.

DRINK UP
Half-fill four serving glasses with the milk kefir and top up with the sparkling or still water. Stir to combine and serve immediately, topped with cotton candy and rose petals, if using. Alternatively, pour the milk kefir into a 1-quart (1 liter) glass jar or bottle with a tight-fitting lid, store in the fridge and top up with the water to serve.

TIP *For an ultrarefreshing and calming drink, add some diced cucumber when serving.*

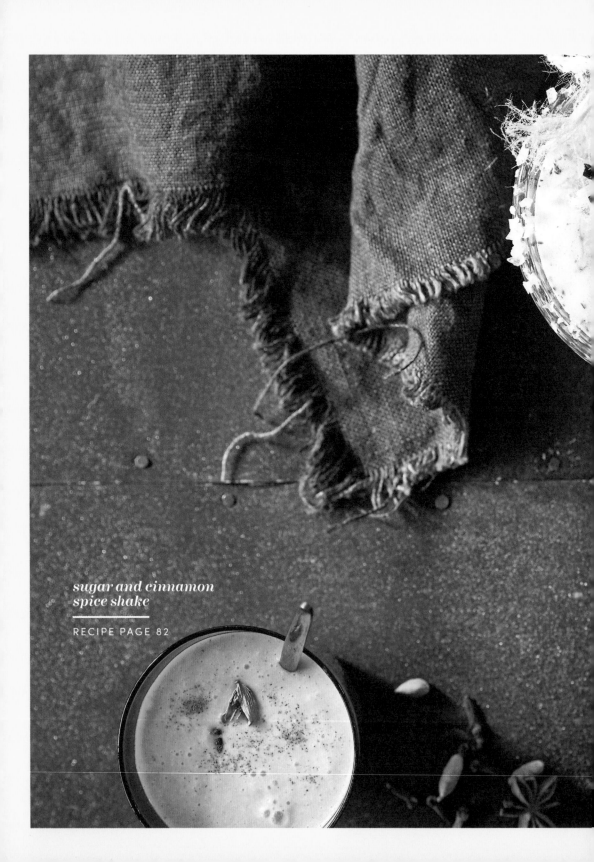

sugar and cinnamon spice shake

RECIPE PAGE 82

Persian mint drink

RECIPE PAGE 83

3. KOMBUCHA

Consumed by monks, grannies and hipsters with equal gusto, kombucha is a popular, easy-to-make, go-to probiotic drink. It's essentially fermented tea – the magic comes when you add the different flavorings and botanics. The first time I drank kombucha was in Mexico, and I was intrigued by the acidic, vinegary but pleasant effervescent flavor. I had never tasted anything like it before. I am an absolute tea connoisseur, so I love kombucha and the opportunity to play around with different teas.

Kombucha is fermented using a SCOBY, which is essentially a collection of yeasts, fungus and bacteria clustered together to form a placenta-like mushroom – but don't let that put you off! The name for this mushroom is a "zoogleal mat" or, colloquially, the "Mother." A kombucha SCOBY is very hardy and easy to manage, and copes well in an acidic environment.

Legend has it that the first use of kombucha was in China in 221 BCE during the Qin Dynasty, where it was known as "the tea of immortality." Kombucha is known by different names in China, Japan, Korea, Vietnam and Russia, but they all translate to "tea fungus" or "tea mushroom."

KOMBUCHA FERMENTATION

There are a number of variables in kombucha fermentation that will affect how long it takes to ferment. These include:

* temperature
* tannins in the tea
* quantity of sugars
* strength of the Mother
* ratio of the Mother to the liquid.

Your kombucha should taste acidic and a little vinegary when you bottle it. If it's too sweet, it needs to ferment longer. Use your intuition and taste preferences as well as the fermentation guidelines and troubleshooting tips on the following pages to guide you.

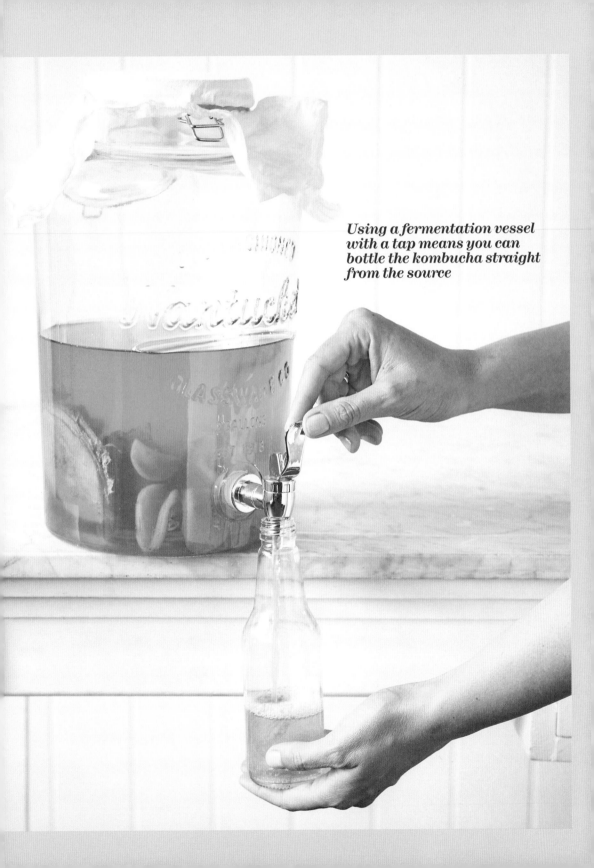

Using a fermentation vessel with a tap means you can bottle the kombucha straight from the source

KOMBUCHA
FERMENTATION GUIDELINES

SCOBY size

You need to purchase or source a kombucha Mother that is around the size of your palm to ferment a 1-quart (1 liter) brew. When the Mother gets bigger than that, you can increase the quantity of tea and honey. A bigger Mother will ferment faster and could turn vinegary much faster. A smaller Mother will take longer to transform the sugar tea.

Starter culture liquid

You should receive the kombucha starter culture liquid when you purchase the Mother. You need ¼ cup (60 ml) starter culture liquid to ferment a 1-quart (1 liter) brew. Once you start brewing, you can use the liquid from a previous brew. Reserve ¼ cup (60 ml) of the kombucha liquid at bottling stage each time you make a brew, ready to use in the next batch. Store the starter culture liquid with the kombucha SCOBY in a container – they should always be kept together as a set.

Tea

If you have a favorite tea that isn't included in the recipes, go ahead and use it. Note that the oils and herbs in flavored tea, such as Earl Grey or herbal tea, may affect the Mother, so you will need to brew your next batch in black or green tea after harvesting the kombucha. If you want to avoid caffeine, use weak tea or decaffeinated tea. The Mother may start to look a little less vigorous, so use caffeinated tea to make up a strong sugar-tea solution (see opposite) and rest the Mother in this solution for 4 to 14 days. The Mother is ready to return to a less caffeinated environment when the liquid tastes slightly acidic and not as sweet as it did when you began.

Sugar

Sugar is the fuel for kombucha and is needed for successful fermentation, so don't scrimp. By the time you drink the kombucha, most of the sugar will have been eaten by the SCOBY, leaving you with a low-sugar elixir. Use only raw or white sugar – don't be tempted to try honey, panela, coconut sugar, molasses or other alternatives. Your SCOBY won't like them.

First fermentation vessel

Use a heatproof 6-cup (1.5 liter) wide-mouth glass or food-grade plastic jar to ferment the kombucha. Metal is no good for kombucha (you can use a metal strainer and utensils). The kombucha Mother will take the shape of the fermentation vessel it's placed in.

Covering

Kombucha is an aerobic fermentation process, so it likes oxygen in the first fermentation stage. Cover the fermentation vessel with a piece of cheesecloth or clean dry dusting cloth and secure it with a rubber band.

During the secondary fermentation, the bottle needs to be tightly sealed with a lid to allow the carbonation to develop.

Bottling

I recommend using a 1-quart (1 liter) sturdy glass bottle with a narrow neck and a tight-fitting lid (similar to a champagne bottle) as this shape will encourage carbonation to develop. The lid needs a good seal so that the fizz stays in the bottle. A bottle with a flip-top rubber stopper is suitable. You will also need a strainer and a funnel.

Position of the Mother during fermentation
The Mother may sink to the bottom of the fermentation vessel. This is fine for the first 3 days or so of fermentation. If it hasn't risen to the surface of the brew after 3 days, you should source a new Mother.

Yeast strands
Strands and floaty bits hanging off the Mother are normal and you can drink these.

Sediment
Some sediment (called "lees") may appear in both the first and second fermentation stages. This is normal. Either stir it up and add it to your finished kombucha, or use it as the starter culture for your next brew.

Reusing or resting the Mother
After bottling, you have two options for the Mother. Either reuse the Mother immediately in your next brew, or rest it in a sugar-tea solution in the fridge (see right).

Rinsing the Mother
Don't rinse the Mother, as this will wash away the good bacteria and yeasts that you are trying to cultivate.

Taking a break from fermentation
The Mother should be fine if it's immersed in a cooled, strong sugar-tea solution (see below) and stored in the fridge for up to 3 months. It may take two to three brews in fresh sugar tea to restore the Mother to vigorous fermentation. These trial brews are fine to bottle and drink if they taste good.

RESTING THE MOTHER

If you go away or want to take a break, you need to rest the Mother in a sugar-tea solution in the fridge.

SUGAR-TEA SOLUTION
1 cup (250 ml) boiling filtered water
4 black tea bags
1 cup (220 g) raw or white sugar
1 cup (250 ml) cold water

Pour the boiling water into a heatproof bowl or teapot and add the tea bags. Steep for 1 minute or so, then discard the tea bags.
    Add the sugar and stir to dissolve. Top up with the cold water.
    Pour the sugar-tea solution into a container and add the kombucha Mother. Seal and place in the fridge for up to 3 months.

HOW TO KNOW WHEN YOUR
KOBUCHA ──
IS READY FOR BOTTLING

SMELL

You should be able to smell the acids of the kombucha as it ferments. The kombucha should have a vinegary, acidic smell. You will definitely notice a change from sweet to sour.

LOOK

You should see small bubbles on the side of the fermentation vessel. You may see bubbles rising up from the bottom of the jar to the top. The Mother should be floating at the top of the vessel and could have a few bubbly, foamy bits.

LISTEN

Generally kombucha fermentation does not have an audible bubbling sound, so tune in to your sense of taste and smell.

TASTE

There should be a lingering tea aroma with a sour and vinegary taste, and sometimes a slight bitter aftertaste. A "young" kombucha will still have sweetness to it, and be very fizzy after secondary fermentation, whereas a "mature" kombucha will taste quite vinegary – but still great to drink!

KOMBUCHA
TROUBLESHOOTING

WHAT IF THE MOTHER ISN'T REPRODUCING?

If the Mother is viable, it should reproduce. A thin transparent film will appear on top of the brew or the Mother – this is the baby SCOBY. Once the film becomes firmer you can peel off the layers, using clean hands, and use them to start a new brew, give them away or leave them together to keep growing. Keep in mind that the thicker the Mother is, the faster fermentation will occur. You need to gradually increase the proportion of tea and the other ingredients, otherwise your kombucha will ferment too quickly and could turn vinegary.

If the Mother doesn't grow a baby, be patient. It may take some time. The growth of a baby is determined by many factors, including:

* temperature
* ingredients
* the age and strength of the Mother
* water quality

WHAT IF THE MOTHER BECOMES MOLDY?

Occasionally you may notice mold growing on the Mother, ranging from white to black and furry. Discard this Mother and the kombucha and source a new Mother.

WHAT IF THE MOTHER IS SINKING?

This is normal for the first 1 to 3 days. If, however, the Mother is still sinking after this time discard the Mother and source a fresh one, as it's possibly not viable.

WHAT IF FERMENTATION ISN'T HAPPENING?

There could be several reasons why the kombucha is not fermenting. Consider the questions below.

Is the Mother sinking? It may not be viable and you may need to source a new one. If the Mother is floating, be patient. In cooler temperatures the kombucha may take up to several weeks to ferment.

Is your water chlorinated? This could inhibit fermentation. Use filtered or spring water for best results.

WHAT IF MY KOMBUCHA IS TOO SOUR?

It was fermented for too long. It's still fine to drink – either as a vinegar shot or with some sweet fruit juice added.

WHAT IF MY KOMBUCHA IS TOO SWEET?

It was harvested too soon. Put it back on to ferment for several days or weeks until it has that distinctive sourness to it.

RECIPES

basic kombucha

In kombucha brewing, the sugars convert into acids, leaving a low-sugar drink. I like to harvest the kombucha when it's still a little sweet. However, if you want to make a vinegar or a totally sugar-free product, allow it to ferment for several weeks and use the kombucha vinegar in salad dressings.

Preparation time: 15 minutes **Fermentation time:** 1–5 weeks **Difficulty:** Medium
Shelf life: Refrigerate for up to 3 months **Makes:** About 1 quart (1 liter)

INGREDIENTS
1 quart (1 liter) filtered water or spring water
4 black tea bags or 1 tablespoon plus 2 teaspoons loose-leaf black tea
¼ cup (55 g) raw or white sugar
¼ cup (60 ml) kombucha starter culture liquid
1 kombucha Mother, a little smaller than the size of your palm

PRIMARY FERMENTATION
Bring 2 cups (500 ml) of the filtered water to a simmer. Pour into a teapot or heatproof bowl, add the tea bags or tea leaves and leave to steep for 3 to 5 minutes. Strain the tea into a heatproof 6-cup (1.5 liter) wide-mouth glass jar and discard the tea bags or tea leaves. Add the sugar to the jar and stir to dissolve. Pour in the remaining filtered water.

When the liquid has cooled to room temperature, add the kombucha starter culture liquid and Mother. Cover the jar with a piece of cheesecloth and secure with a rubber band.

Place the jar out of direct sunlight in a cool spot where it won't be disturbed. Leave the liquid to ferment for around 4 days in hot weather and 14 to 20 days in cooler weather.

BOTTLING

Gently remove the Mother to reuse or rest (see page 89).
Retain ¼ cup (60 ml) of the kombucha liquid as the starter
culture liquid for your next brew (see page 88).

Mix in any sediment that has settled at the bottom of the
jar, or leave it as it is. Put a funnel in the opening of a 1-quart
(1 liter) glass bottle with a tight-fitting lid and put a strainer
on top of the funnel. Pour the kombucha into the bottle
through the strainer and discard any solids.

SECONDARY FERMENTATION

Tightly seal the bottle lid and leave the bottle on the counter
to build carbonation. This could take anywhere from 2 to 14
days, depending on the temperature. "Burp" the kombucha
daily to release some pressure by opening the lid slightly
and then tightening it again.

DRINK UP

When the kombucha is as fizzy and sour as you like (this
could range from a small spritz to a ferocious fizz), store it in
the fridge to slow the fermentation process, and enjoy cold.

TIP   *You can make a fabulous hair rinse from kombucha
that will leave your hair soft and silky. Allow fermentation
to continue to vinegar stage, so that no sugar is left – the
kombucha will smell highly acidic. Bottle the kombucha
and use it next time you wash your hair.*

Earl Grey kombucha with lemon

The defining feature of Earl Grey tea is the addition of bergamot oil, which is the cold-pressed oil from inside the rind of the bergamot orange. The bergamot orange is known as "sour orange," which tastes more bitter than a grapefruit but less sour than a lemon. Apparently Earl Grey tea was created to mimic the more expensive types of Chinese tea, and has been used in England since the 1820s.

Preparation time: 15 minutes **Fermentation time:** 1–5 weeks **Difficulty:** Medium
Shelf life: Refrigerate for up to 3 months **Makes:** About 1 quart (1 liter)

INGREDIENTS
1 recipe basic kombucha
(page 92); replace the black
tea with Earl Grey tea
½ lemon

PRIMARY FERMENTATION
Follow the instructions for basic kombucha, using Earl Grey tea instead of black tea.

BOTTLING
Follow the instructions for basic kombucha.

SECONDARY FERMENTATION
Squeeze the lemon juice into the bottle and tightly seal the lid. Leave the bottle on the counter to build carbonation. This could take anywhere from 2 to 14 days, depending on the temperature. "Burp" the kombucha daily to release some pressure by opening the lid slightly and then tightening it again.

DRINK UP
When the kombucha is as fizzy and sour as you like (this could range from a small spritz to a ferocious fizz), store it in the fridge to slow the fermentation process, and enjoy cold.

TIP *The bergamot oils in fragrant Earl Grey could, over time, decrease the effectiveness of the Mother. I recommend using this recipe when you have a back-up Mother. It's best to rotate this kombucha with the basic kombucha (see page 92) that uses black tea.*

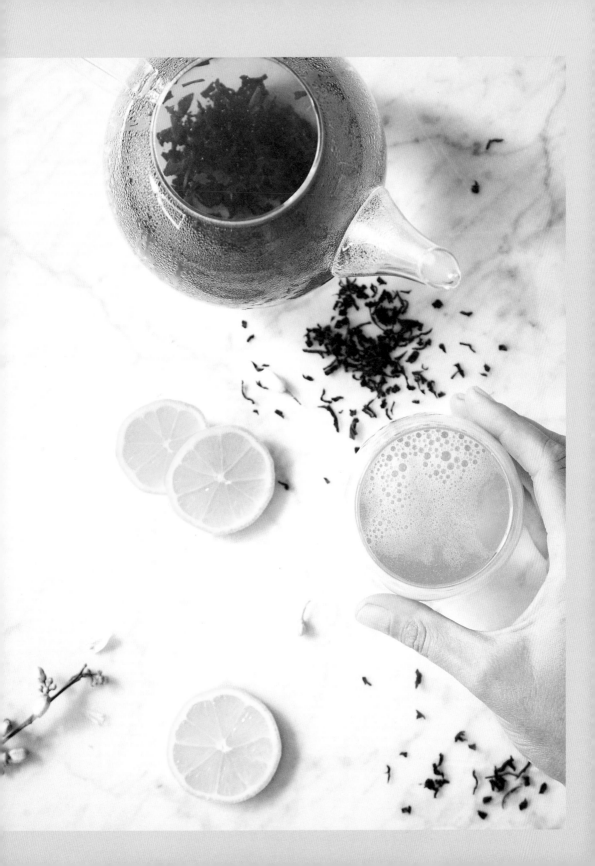

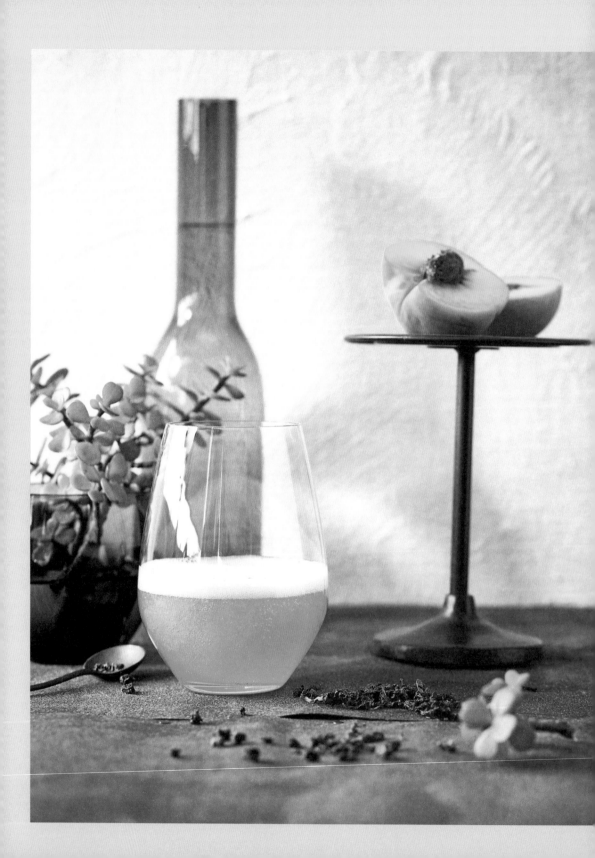

oolong kombucha with fragrant peach

Oolong tea is halfway between green tea and black tea, and the color and taste is a combination of the two. Leaves for oolong tea are picked early in the day and fermented. Once fermentation is complete, the tea leaves are rubbed, which releases the aroma and flavor. Finally, the leaves are dried and packaged. This version of kombucha makes a milder, fruitier and grassy-tasting kombucha.

Preparation time: 15 minutes **Fermentation time:** 1–5 weeks **Difficulty:** Medium
Shelf life: Refrigerate for up to 3 months **Makes:** About 1 quart (1 liter)

INGREDIENTS

*1 recipe basic kombucha
(page 92); replace the black
tea with oolong tea
1 ripe peach, chopped, or ½ cup
(125 ml) peach nectar
(see Tip)*

PRIMARY FERMENTATION

Follow the instructions for basic kombucha, using oolong tea instead of black tea.

BOTTLING

Follow the instructions for basic kombucha.

SECONDARY FERMENTATION

Add the chopped peach or peach nectar to the bottle and tightly seal the lid. Leave the bottle on the counter to build carbonation. This could take anywhere from 2 to 14 days, depending on the temperature. "Burp" the kombucha daily to release some pressure by opening the lid slightly and then tightening it again.

DRINK UP

When the kombucha is as fizzy and sour as you like (this could range from a small spritz to a ferocious fizz), store it in the fridge to slow the fermentation process, and enjoy cold.

TIP *If you can't find peach nectar, use any stone fruit or nectar you can find – the results will be similar.*

white tea kombucha with guava nectar

White tea is considered one of the finest of all teas and for some connoisseurs it is the pinnacle of sophistication and perfection. Even though it comes from the same plant as more common black tea, it's not rolled and oxidized, so it has a lighter taste. White tea is packed with antioxidants and polyphenols and has a sweet but subtle flavor. The guava nectar adds a lovely rounding to the lightness of the kombucha, but this variety is also gorgeous on its own, without the guava.

Preparation time: 15 minutes **Fermentation time:** 1–5 weeks **Difficulty:** Medium
Shelf life: Refrigerate for up to 3 months **Makes:** About 1 quart (1 liter)

INGREDIENTS
1 recipe basic kombucha (page 92); replace the black tea with white tea
½ cup (125 ml) guava nectar

PRIMARY FERMENTATION
Follow the instructions for basic kombucha, using white tea instead of black tea.

BOTTLING
Follow the instructions for basic kombucha.

SECONDARY FERMENTATION
Add the guava nectar to the bottle and tightly seal the lid. Leave the bottle on the counter to build carbonation. This could take anywhere from 2 to 14 days, depending on the temperature. "Burp" the kombucha daily to release some pressure by opening the lid slightly and then tightening it again.

DRINK UP
When the kombucha is as fizzy and sour as you like (this could range from a small spritz to a ferocious fizz), store it in the fridge to slow the fermentation process, and enjoy cold.

green tea kombucha with apple

This kombucha is a beautiful way to bottle up and enjoy all the powerful antioxidants found in green tea. The apple adds a lovely crisp and refreshing finish to this elixir. Experiment with different apple varieties from your local farmers' market.

Preparation time: 15 minutes **Fermentation time:** 1–5 weeks **Difficulty:** Medium
Shelf life: Refrigerate for up to 3 months **Makes:** About 1 quart (1 liter)

INGREDIENTS

1 recipe basic kombucha (page 92); replace the black tea with green tea
1 apple, chopped, or ½ cup (125 ml) apple juice

PRIMARY FERMENTATION

Follow the instructions for basic kombucha, using green tea instead of black tea.

BOTTLING

Follow the instructions for basic kombucha.

SECONDARY FERMENTATION

Add the chopped apple or apple juice to the bottle and tightly seal the lid. Leave the bottle on the counter to build carbonation. This could take anywhere from 2 to 14 days, depending on the temperature. "Burp" the kombucha daily to release some pressure by opening the lid slightly and then tightening it again.

DRINK UP

When the kombucha is as fizzy and sour as you like (this could range from a small spritz to a ferocious fizz), store it in the fridge to slow the fermentation process, and enjoy cold.

VARIATION *Add 2 dried elderberries to the bottle along with the apple for a lovely elderberry flavor.*

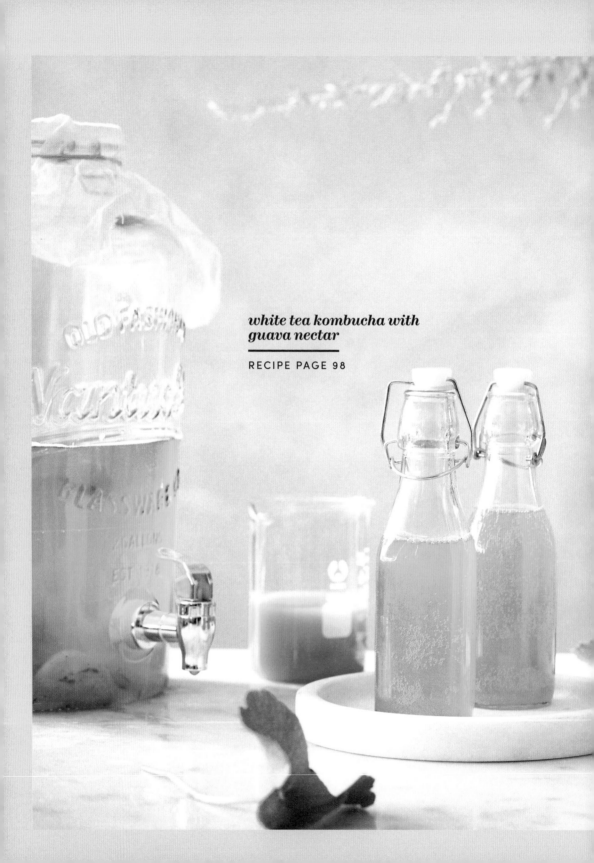

*white tea kombucha with
guava nectar*

RECIPE PAGE 98

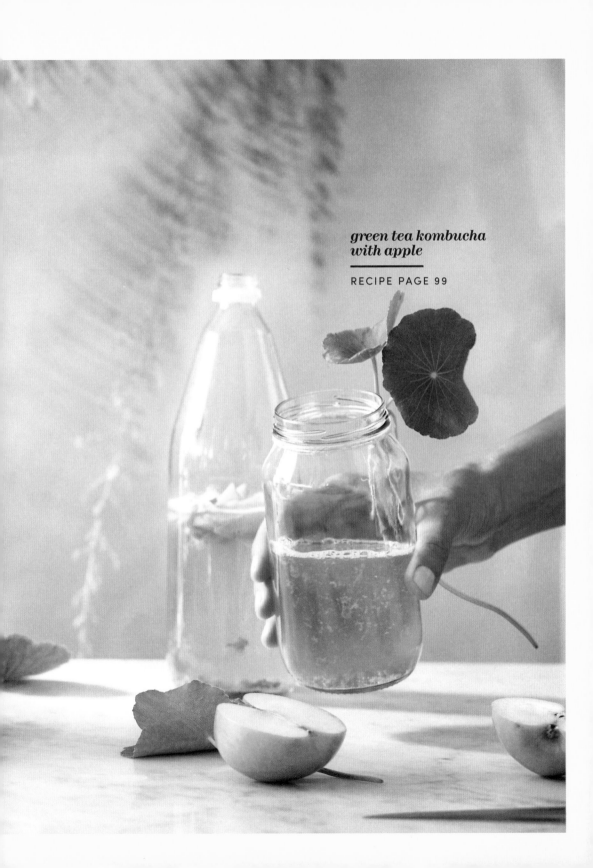

*green tea kombucha
with apple*

RECIPE PAGE 99

striking rooibos and hibiscus kombucha

———

This kombucha is perfect if you're avoiding caffeine and want to add more herbal goodness to your diet. Rooibos is a South African herb, which contains antioxidants and minerals, including magnesium, calcium, manganese, zinc and iron. Hibiscus is a tart and astringent herb with a gorgeous crimson color. The Mother may take on the color of the hibiscus and turn pink.

Preparation time: 15 minutes **Fermentation time:** 1–5 weeks **Difficulty:** Medium
Shelf life: Refrigerate for up to 3 months **Makes:** About 1 quart (1 liter)

———

INGREDIENTS
1 recipe basic kombucha (page 92); replace the black tea with rooibos tea
2 hibiscus tea bags or 2 teaspoons loose-leaf hibiscus tea

PRIMARY FERMENTATION
Follow the instructions for basic kombucha, using rooibos and hibiscus teas instead of black tea.

BOTTLING
Follow the instructions for basic kombucha.

SECONDARY FERMENTATION
Tightly seal the bottle lid and leave the bottle on the counter to build carbonation. This could take anywhere from 2 to 14 days, depending on the temperature. "Burp" the kombucha daily to release some pressure by opening the lid slightly and then tightening it again.

DRINK UP
When the kombucha is as fizzy and sour as you like (this could range from a small spritz to a ferocious fizz), store it in the fridge to slow the fermentation process, and enjoy cold.

———

TIP *If you don't have access to hibiscus tea, you can omit it. Or, if you want the crimson color, use finely chopped ripe plums, strawberries or raspberries. Add them to the kombucha at the bottling stage.*

———

botanical elixir kombucha

Capture and preserve the calming and restorative qualities of rosemary and lavender in this sensual and relaxing plant-infused elixir. Rosemary has traditionally been used to help relax muscle pain and promote hair growth. Lavender has a gorgeous perfume and is used to help relieve anxiety.

Preparation time: 15 minutes **Fermentation time:** 1–5 weeks **Difficulty:** Medium
Shelf life: Refrigerate for up to 3 months **Makes:** About 1 quart (1 liter)

INGREDIENTS

1 recipe basic kombucha (page 92); replace the black tea with green tea
1 lavender sprig
1 rosemary sprig

PRIMARY FERMENTATION

Follow the instructions for basic kombucha, using green tea instead of black tea.

BOTTLING

Follow the instructions for basic kombucha.

SECONDARY FERMENTATION

Add the lavender and rosemary sprigs to the bottle and tightly seal the lid. Leave the bottle on the counter to build carbonation. This could take anywhere from 2 to 14 days, depending on the temperature. "Burp" the kombucha daily to release some pressure by opening the lid slightly and then tightening it again.

DRINK UP

When the kombucha is as fizzy and sour as you like (this could range from a small spritz to a ferocious fizz), store it in the fridge to slow the fermentation process, and enjoy cold.

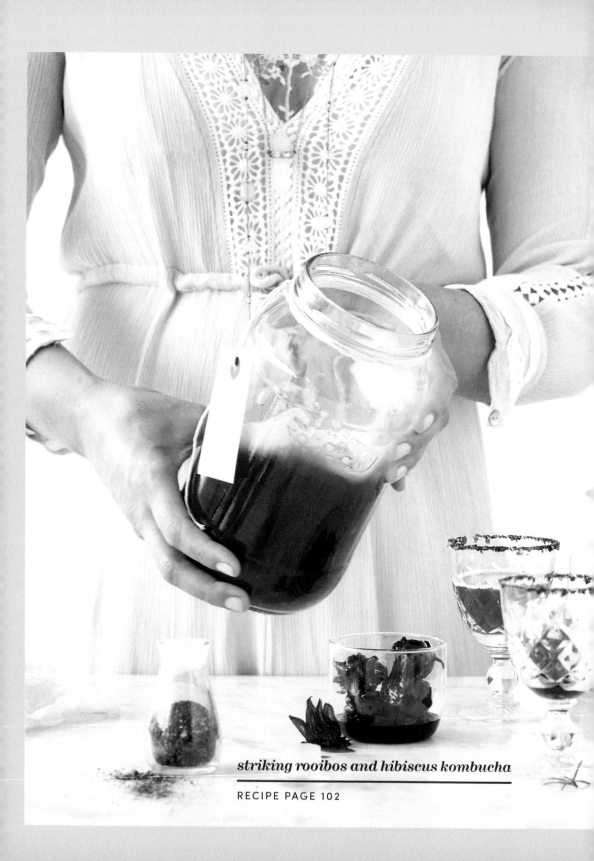

striking rooibos and hibiscus kombucha

RECIPE PAGE 102

botanical elixir kombucha

RECIPE PAGE 103

4. JUN

Jun is an effervescent fermented tea and is known as the "champagne of kombuchas" for its light and bubbly taste. It has a similar fermentation process and appearance to kombucha. However, while kombucha has a strong, distinctive taste, Jun is softer and lighter, with a more delicate taste. The roundness of the honey notes makes the flavor full and buttery. Jun is packed with living probiotics and antioxidants from the green tea that it ferments.

Jun makes a stunning aperitif, cleansing the palate and getting the digestive enzymes into gear in anticipation of a beautiful meal. It can produce an alcohol content of around 2 percent, so you may want to dilute it with soda water.

The Jun SCOBY is a soft, padded disk that looks like a kombucha SCOBY, but it is unique because it ferments only green tea and honey. It's like a blend of honey mead and kombucha, but don't be fooled – Jun is not masquerading as kombucha. It's an entirely different culture and has a different fermentation process, with a shorter fermentation time, and it prefers cooler temperatures.

There are very few known facts about Jun's origin and history. Legend has it that monks and warriors used Jun for centuries in the cool climate of the Himalayas, where it was brewed in order to aid enlightenment.

There is a reverence around Jun and it's believed that Lao Tzu, the ancient Chinese philosopher and writer of the *Tao Te Ching*, gave an heirloom culture to the monks of Bon in Tibet. This may just be a story, because the history and origins of Jun are shrouded in mystery and secrecy. That's one of the reasons I love Jun so much.

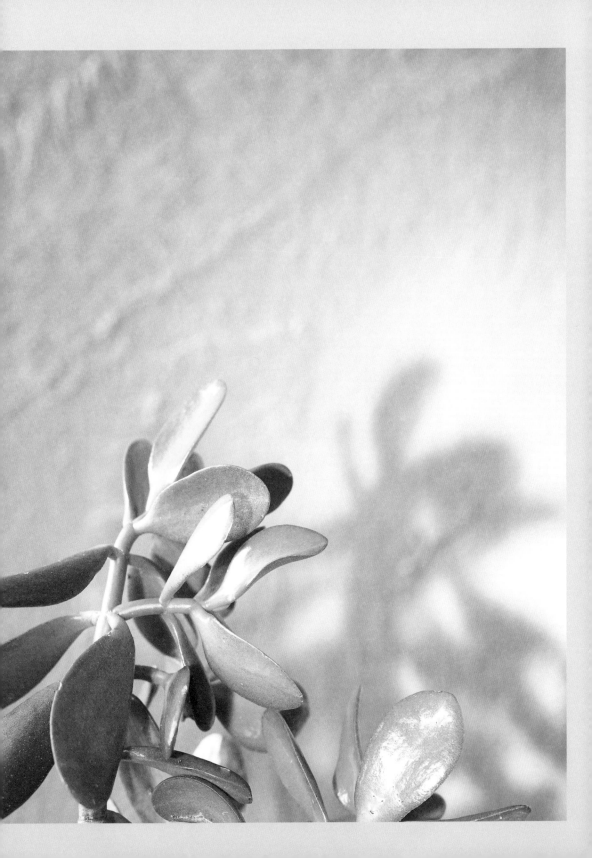

FERMENTATION GUIDELINES

SCOBY size

The Jun SCOBY you need to ferment a 1-quart (1 liter) brew is around the size of your palm. When the SCOBY gets bigger than that, you can double the quantity of tea and honey. A bigger SCOBY will probably ferment faster and could turn vinegary much faster. A smaller SCOBY will take a lot longer to transform the honey green tea. The Jun SCOBY is more delicate and slower to grow compared with kombucha, even though they look very similar, so you need to be patient. It prefers to not be handled too much.

Starter culture liquid

You should receive the Jun starter culture liquid when you purchase the Jun SCOBY. You need ¼ cup (60 ml) starter culture liquid to ferment a 1-quart (1 liter) brew. Once you start brewing, you can use the liquid from a previous brew. Reserve ¼ cup (60 ml) of the Jun liquid at bottling stage each time you make a brew, ready to use in the next batch. Store the Jun starter culture liquid with the Jun SCOBY in a container – they should always be kept together as a set.

Tea

Jun is distinct in that it ferments green tea only, so don't use other types of tea as it will ruin the Jun SCOBY. Choose the best quality organic green tea you can find. Loose tea leaves or tea bags are fine.

Honey

The quality of the honey you use will directly affect the quality and taste of your Jun. For best results, use raw honey. I prefer to use a lighter tasting honey as the final flavor is softer.

First fermentation vessel

Use a 6-cup (1.5 liter) wide-mouth glass or food-grade plastic jar to ferment the Jun. Metal is no good for Jun (you can use a metal strainer and utensils).

Covering

Jun is an aerobic fermentation process, so it likes oxygen in the first fermentation stage. Cover the fermentation vessel with a piece of cheesecloth or clean dry dusting cloth and secure it with a rubber band.

Bottling

I recommend using a 1-quart (1 liter) sturdy glass bottle with a narrow neck and a tight-fitting lid (similar to a champagne bottle) as this shape will encourage carbonation to develop. The lid needs a good seal so that the fizz stays in the bottle. A bottle with a flip-top rubber stopper is suitable. You will also need a strainer and a funnel.

Position of the SCOBY during fermentation

The Jun SCOBY should float during the fermentation process. If it sinks and doesn't seem to ferment the honey tea, you will need to source a new SCOBY.

Sediment

Some sediment (called "lees") may appear in both the first and second fermentation stages. This is normal. Either stir it up and add it to your finished Jun, or use it as the starter culture for your next brew.

Reusing or resting the SCOBY

After bottling, you have two options for the Jun SCOBY. Either reuse the SCOBY immediately in your next brew, or rest the SCOBY in a green tea and honey solution in the fridge (see right).

Rinsing the SCOBY

Don't rinse the Jun SCOBY, as this will wash away the good bacteria and yeasts that you are trying to cultivate.

Taking a break from fermentation

The SCOBY should be fine if it's immersed in a cooled green tea and honey solution (see right) and stored in the fridge for up to 3 months. It may take two to three brews in fresh honey tea to restore the SCOBY to vigorous fermentation. These trial brews are fine to bottle and drink if they taste good.

RESTING THE SCOBY

If you go away, or have an excess of culture, you need to rest the Jun SCOBY in a green tea and honey solution in the fridge.

GREEN TEA AND HONEY SOLUTION

1 cup (250 ml) boiling filtered water
4 green tea bags
¼ cup (85 g) raw honey

Pour the boiling water into a large mug and add the tea bags. Steep for 40 to 60 seconds, then discard the tea bags.

Add the honey and stir to dissolve. Leave to cool to room temperature.

Pour the green tea and honey solution into a glass container and add the Jun SCOBY. Cover with a loose-fitting lid and place in the fridge for up to 3 months.

HOW TO KNOW WHEN YOUR
JUN
IS READY FOR BOTTLING

SMELL

Finished Jun should have a slight vinegary smell. It won't smell sweet and honey-like – it will be a little more acidic. You will definitely notice a change from sweet to sour. You may also experience a yeasty hit when you first smell the finished product. This is a good sign that fermentation has taken place.

LOOK

You should see some small bubbles on the side of the fermentation vessel. You may also see bubbles rising up from the bottom of the jar. This is active fermentation in motion! It's completely normal to see sediment fall to the bottom of the fermentation vessel. I usually filter this out when bottling.

LISTEN

There is not a strong fizzing sound as Jun ferments. If anything, there will be a very slight bubbling sound.

TASTE

Jun has an unusual and delicate fizzy taste. It's savory and not sugar-sweet. The addition of the honey rounds out the flavor, making it cleansing and light. There is a little bit of an acidic/ vinegary taste. When you first start fermenting, I recommend tasting the Jun every couple of days so that you learn to understand how the ferment changes over time.

TROUBLESHOOTING

WHAT IF THE SCOBY ISN'T REPRODUCING?

The Jun SCOBY is generally slow to reproduce, so be patient. If the SCOBY is viable, it should reproduce. A thin transparent film will appear on top of the brew or the SCOBY – this is the baby SCOBY. Once the film becomes firmer you can peel off the layers, using clean hands, and use them to start a new brew, give them away or leave them together to keep growing. Keep in mind that the thicker the SCOBY is, the faster fermentation will occur. You need to gradually increase the proportion of tea and the other ingredients, otherwise your Jun will ferment too quickly and could turn vinegary.

If the SCOBY doesn't grow a baby, be patient. It may take some time. The growth of a baby SCOBY is determined by many factors, including:

    temperature
    ingredients
    the age and strength of the SCOBY
    water quality.

WHAT IF THE SCOBY BECOMES MOLDY?

Occasionally you may notice mold growing on the SCOBY, ranging from white to black. Discard this SCOBY and the Jun and source a new SCOBY.

WHAT IF MY JUN IS TOO VINEGARY?

If the Jun is too vinegary with a strong smell, it was fermented for too long. It's still fine to drink, but you may want to sweeten it a little, or drink it as a tonic rather than a fizzy drink.

WHAT IF MY JUN IS TOO SWEET?

It was harvested too soon. Put it back on to ferment for longer.

RECIPES

basic Jun

The quality of the green tea and honey you choose will affect the final taste, so choose the best quality you can afford. I always use organic green tea and raw honey so that the Jun culture and I both get the best quality available and there are no pesticides that could kill the good bacteria.

Preparation time: 30 minutes **Fermentation time:** 6–17 days **Difficulty:** Easy–medium
Shelf life: Refrigerate for up to 4 months **Makes:** About 1 quart (1 liter)

INGREDIENTS
1 quart (1 liter) filtered water or spring water
4 green tea bags or 1 tablespoon plus 1 teaspoon loose-leaf green tea
¼ cup (85 g) raw honey
¼ cup (60 ml) Jun starter culture liquid
1 Jun SCOBY, around the size of your palm

PRIMARY FERMENTATION
Bring 2 cups (500 ml) of the filtered water to a simmer. Pour into a teapot or heatproof bowl, add the green tea bags or tea leaves and leave to steep for 40 to 60 seconds. Strain the tea into a heatproof 1-quart (1.5 liter) wide-mouth glass jar and discard the tea bags or tea leaves. Pour in the remaining water. Add the honey to the jar and stir well to dissolve.

When the liquid has cooled to room temperature, add the Jun starter culture liquid and SCOBY. Cover the jar with a piece of cheesecloth and secure with a rubber band.

Place the jar out of direct sunlight in a cool spot where it won't be disturbed. Leave the liquid to ferment for around 4 days in hot weather and 7 to 10 days in cooler weather.

BOTTLING

Gently remove the SCOBY to reuse or rest (see page 109), and retain ¼ cup (60 ml) of the Jun liquid as the starter culture liquid for your next brew (see page 108).

Mix in any sediment that has settled at the bottom of the jar. Put a funnel in the opening of a 1-quart (1 liter) glass bottle with a tight-fitting lid and put a strainer on top of the funnel. Pour the Jun into the bottle through the strainer. Either discard any solids left in the strainer or incorporate them into your next brew.

SECONDARY FERMENTATION

Tightly seal the bottle lid and leave the bottle on the counter to build carbonation. This could take anywhere from 2 to 7 days, depending on the temperature. "Burp" the Jun daily to release some pressure by opening the lid slightly and then tightening it again.

DRINK UP

When the Jun is as fizzy and sour as you like (this could range from a small spritz to a ferocious fizz), store it in the fridge to slow the fermentation process, and enjoy cold.

———

TIP *Letting green tea steep for too long causes it to turn bitter. Only steep the tea for 40 to 60 seconds.*

———

Jun with jasmine tea

I love the ferments that give you the benefit of the herb or tea as well as the living probiotics. Jasmine flowers add a delicate flowery scent and flavor to Jun. Don't get them confused with the beautiful spring blossoms you may have growing in your garden. There are actually around two hundred species of jasmine, but the one that's cultivated and used in green tea is *Jasminum sambac* or "Arabian jasmine" (even though it's not native to Arabia). *Jasminum sambac* is the national flower of the Philippines and one of three national flowers of Indonesia, and it's also used in perfumes.

Preparation time: 30 minutes **Fermentation time:** 6–17 days **Difficulty:** Easy–medium
Shelf life: Refrigerate for up to 4 months **Makes:** About 1 quart (1 liter)

INGREDIENTS
*1 recipe basic Jun (page 112);
replace the green tea with
jasmine green tea*

PRIMARY FERMENTATION
Follow the instructions for basic Jun, using jasmine green tea instead of green tea.

BOTTLING
Follow the instructions for basic Jun.

SECONDARY FERMENTATION
Tightly seal the bottle lid and leave the bottle on the counter to build carbonation. This could take anywhere from 2 to 7 days, depending on the temperature. "Burp" the Jun daily to release some pressure by opening the lid slightly and then tightening it again.

DRINK UP
When the Jun is as fizzy and sour as you like (this could range from a small spritz to a ferocious fizz), store it in the fridge to slow the fermentation process, and enjoy cold.

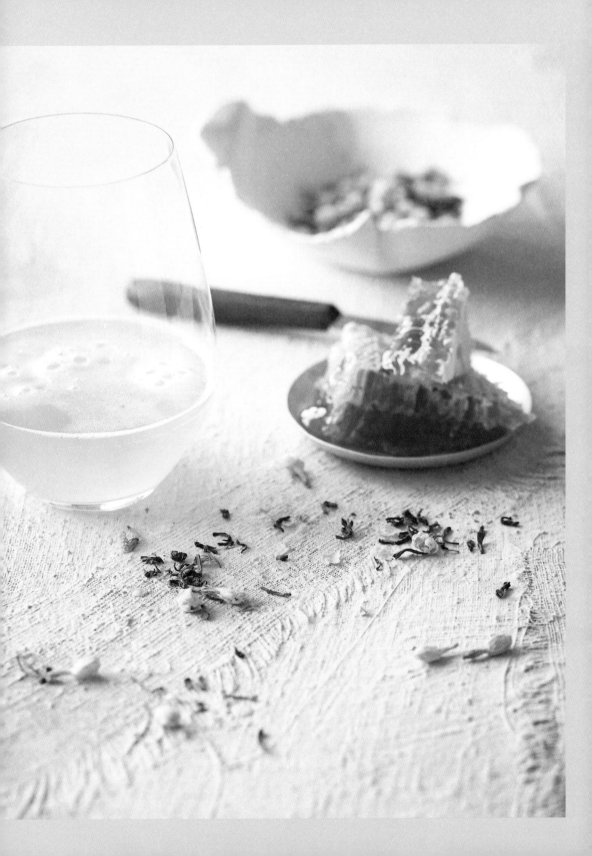

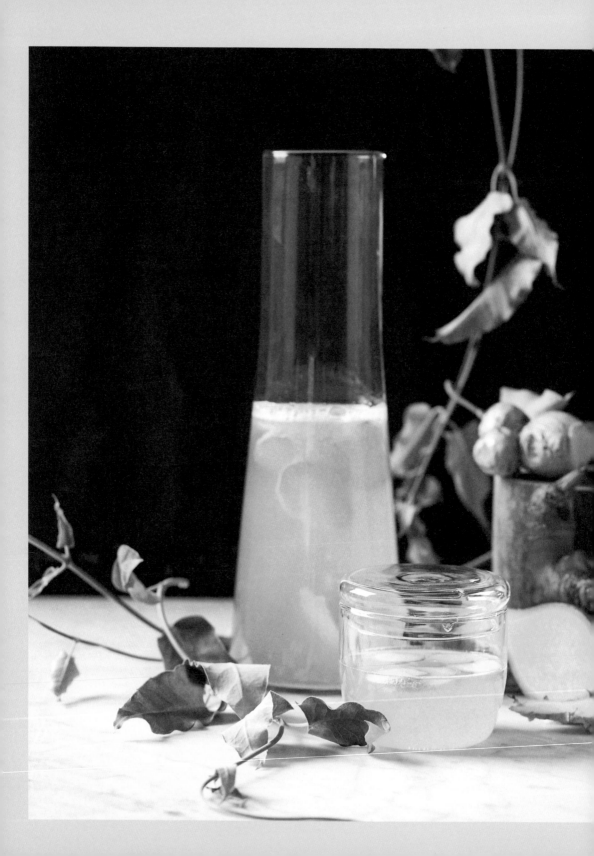

Jun with ginger and galangal

Ginger and galangal pair well with the sweet honey notes in the Jun. They can boost circulation and heat the body, calm nausea and aid in digestion. These two rhizomes complement each other well in the flavor department. Ginger has more of a fiery, pungent and sharp taste, whereas galangal is more peppery and aromatic, with tones of pine. The bacteria and yeasts tend to love the ginger and galangal – you will see lots of carbonation building around the rhizomes. If you don't have both ginger and galangal, just use whichever one you have.

Preparation time: 30 minutes **Fermentation time:** 6–17 days **Difficulty:** Easy–medium
Shelf life: Refrigerate for up to 4 months **Makes:** About 1 quart (1 liter)

INGREDIENTS
1 recipe basic Jun (page 112)
¾-inch (2 cm) piece fresh ginger, skin on, thinly sliced
¾-inch (2 cm) piece fresh galangal, skin on, thinly sliced

PRIMARY FERMENTATION
Follow the instructions for basic Jun.

BOTTLING
Follow the instructions for basic Jun.

SECONDARY FERMENTATION
Add the ginger and galangal to the bottle and tightly seal the lid. Leave the bottle on the counter to build carbonation. This could take anywhere from 2 to 7 days, depending on the temperature. "Burp" the Jun daily to release some pressure by opening the lid slightly and then tightening it again.

DRINK UP
When the Jun is as fizzy and sour as you like (this could range from a small spritz to a ferocious fizz), store it in the fridge to slow the fermentation process, and enjoy cold.

TIPS *You can add more ginger and galangal if you prefer stronger flavors.*
Add a squeeze of sweet and fragrant lime juice when serving the Jun.

Jun with raspberries

Raspberries are the ultimate signal that summer has arrived. If you manage to snatch up excess berries from your local farmers' market, make a big batch of this Jun and enjoy the summer flavor long after the season has finished. Raspberries contain high amounts of antioxidants, phytochemicals and vitamin C, and they're also low GI. When you ferment them, the nutrients are partially broken down in the process, making them easier for your body to absorb. They're an all-round winner.

Preparation time: 30 minutes **Fermentation time:** 6–17 days **Difficulty:** Easy–medium
Shelf life: Refrigerate for up to 4 months **Makes:** About 1 quart (1 liter)

INGREDIENTS
1 recipe basic Jun (page 112)
*¼ cup (30 g) fresh or frozen
  raspberries*

PRIMARY FERMENTATION
Follow the instructions for basic Jun.

BOTTLING
Follow the instructions for basic Jun.

SECONDARY FERMENTATION
Blitz the raspberries in a food processor and add the pulp to the bottle, or simply add the whole raspberries to the bottle. Tightly seal the bottle lid and leave the bottle on the counter to build carbonation. This could take anywhere from 2 to 7 days, depending on the temperature. "Burp" the Jun daily to release some pressure by opening the lid slightly and then tightening it again.

DRINK UP
When the Jun is as fizzy and sour as you like (this could range from a small spritz to a ferocious fizz), store it in the fridge to slow the fermentation process, and enjoy cold.

TIP *If you have a glut of raspberries (lucky you!), freeze them so you have them on hand all year round to add to your Jun.*

Jun with passionfruit

I have a tradition of giving a passionfruit to friends on special days, such as birthdays, engagement parties and weddings, as a symbol to remind them to add passion to their day. Tacky, perhaps, but definitely memorable! Passionfruit is actually very simple to grow at home if you live in a warmish climate. Take the seeds of a bought passionfruit and put them in a pot with some good soil. Add some water and sunshine and you will have a passionfruit vine in no time.

Preparation time: 30 minutes **Fermentation time:** 6–17 days **Difficulty:** Easy–medium
Shelf life: Refrigerate for up to 4 months **Makes:** About 1 quart (1 liter)

INGREDIENTS
1 recipe basic Jun (page 112)
1 passionfruit

PRIMARY FERMENTATION
Follow the instructions for basic Jun.

BOTTLING
Follow the instructions for basic Jun.

SECONDARY FERMENTATION
Cut the passionfruit in half and spoon the pulp into the bottle. Tightly seal the bottle lid and leave the bottle on the counter to build carbonation. This could take anywhere from 2 to 7 days, depending on the temperature. "Burp" the Jun daily to release some pressure by opening the lid slightly and then tightening it again.

DRINK UP
When the Jun is as fizzy and sour as you like (this could range from a small spritz to a ferocious fizz), store it in the fridge to slow the fermentation process, and enjoy cold.

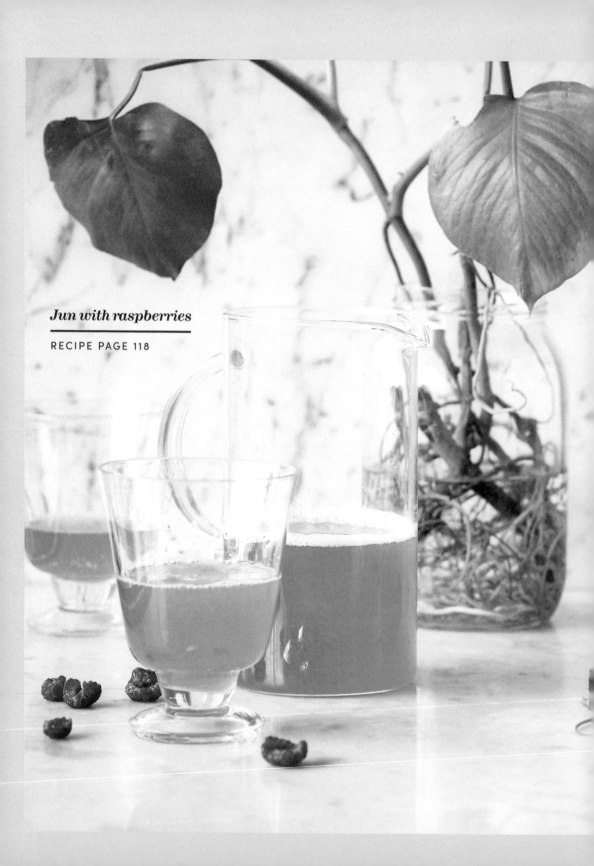

Jun with raspberries

RECIPE PAGE 118

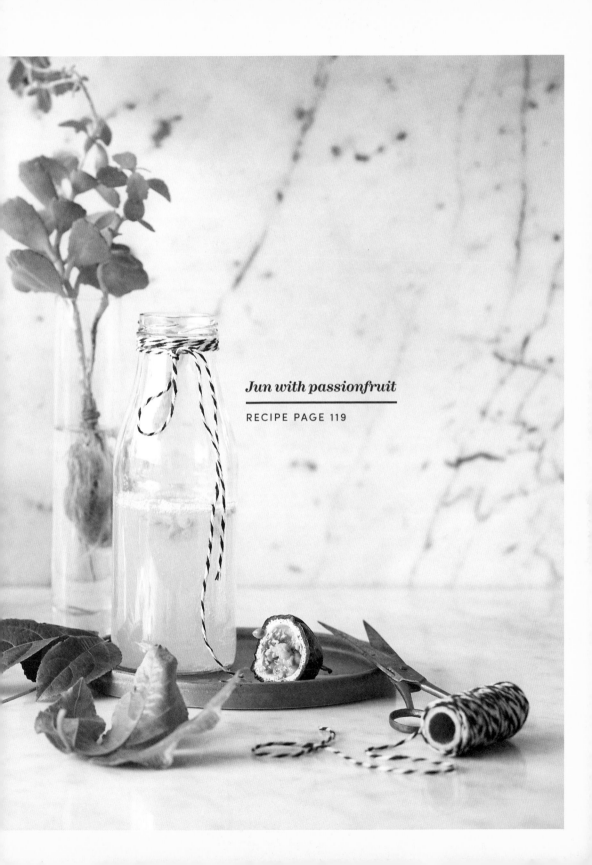

Jun with passionfruit

RECIPE PAGE 119

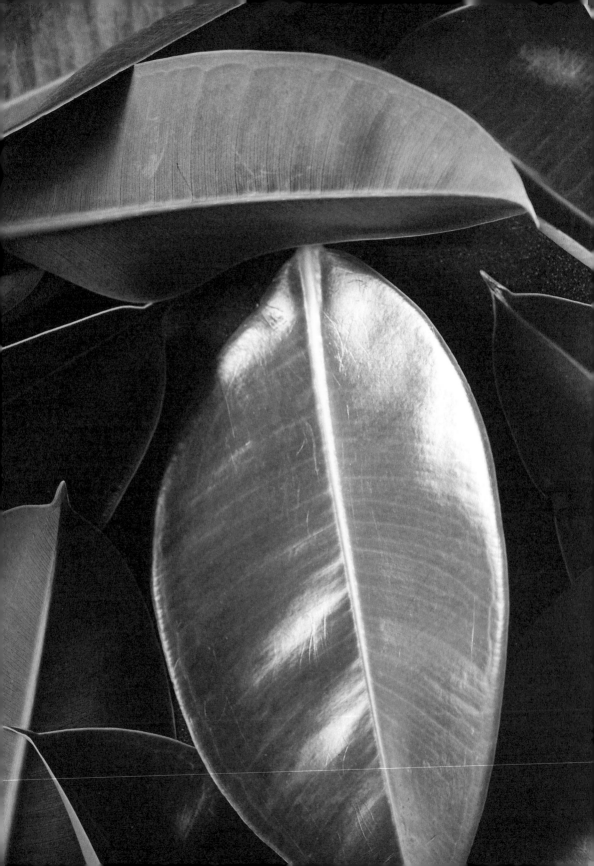

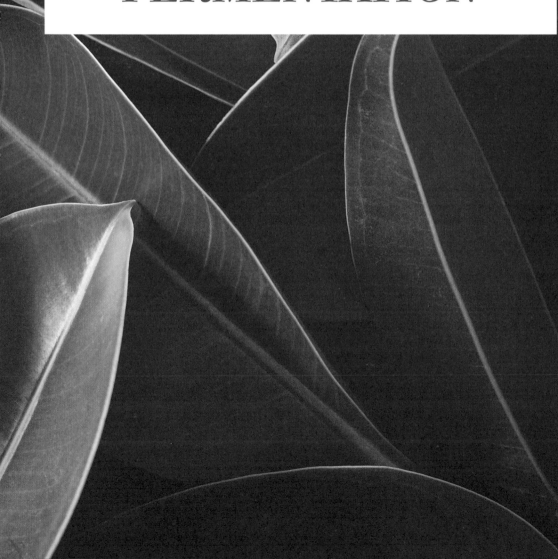

section two

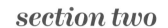

WILD FERMENTATION

INTRODUCTION

In wild fermentation, we harness the wild yeasts and bacteria that live in the air and on the skins of fruits, vegetables and roots to spontaneously start the fermentation process. This wild fermentation can happen with or without human interaction, but for the purposes of this book we will help it along.

In nature, spontaneous wild fermentation happens to sugar-rich fruits when the yeasts and bacteria that are in the air and on the skins of the fruits start to metabolize the sugars and convert them to alcohol and lactic acid. This is true spontaneous wild fermentation.

To make the wild ferments in this book, we help nature along by adding select ingredients and stirring to encourage aeration. For example, in making the ginger bug for ginger beer, we combine fresh ginger with some sugar and a little water. Next we allow the wild yeasts and bacteria from the air to start the fermentation process. The effect of this is that the ginger and sugar-water mixture begins to bubble as fermentation kicks off. That bubbling mixture becomes the starter "bug" for ginger beer.

EXAMPLES OF FERMENTS THAT CAN RELY ON WILD FERMENTATION

* Cocoa
* Coffee
* Tea
* Kvass
* Tepache
* Ginger beer
* Honey mead
* Apple cider
* Sauerkraut
* Kimchi
* Cheeses

SUCCESSFUL AND UNSUCCESSFUL FERMENTATION

Everyone has a different taste profile and tolerance for fermented products, which could be cultural preferences or acquired tastes. For example, some people find the very strong smell and sharp taste of blue cheese highly appealing, while others, not accustomed to the pungency of this ferment, balk at the thought of eating it.

It is important to draw a distinction between "good" wild fermentation and decomposition. There is a continuum along the fermented drinks scale from a beautiful acidic sour flavor and smell, to a drink that is rotten and unsuitable for consumption. Please be aware of this, and err on the side of caution. Refer to the fermentation guidelines and troubleshooting notes in each recipe chapter for helpful tips and advice.

The table below shows the difference between "good" wild fermentation and wild fermentation that is unsafe to drink.

	SUCCESSFUL FERMENTATION	QUESTIONABLE FERMENTATION
SMELL	The smell will be sour and a little acidic, but may also have some sweetness. It may smell "different" from what you would usually smell, but it won't be off-putting.	The smell will be very off-putting, like something rotten that you wouldn't want to eat. This happens when the good bacteria don't have enough food to eat and they die off, giving the destructive bacteria a chance to start decomposition.
TASTE	The taste will be a little sour and a little yeasty.	The taste will be too pungent and musty – you would know not to drink it!
LOOK	There could be little bubbles forming as it ferments.	There could be white or black mold on the surface and it could look a little slimy.

5. BEET KVASS

Beet kvass is an acquired taste. It's salty and earthy, with little sweetness, so it's a great drink if you want to avoid sugars in your diet. It's essentially an infusion of beets, salt and water, fermented by wild yeasts in the air. If you want a daily probiotic shot to keep you in tip-top shape, go for kvass.

Beet kvass is sometimes thought of as a gut tonic and digestive aid. It has fantastic liver-purifying benefits, with a high concentration of beets in a small glass. It's also blood purifying and super nutritive, as the fermentation process increases the availability of the nutrients in the beetroot.

Beet kvass is a multitasking probiotic. It's beautiful as a shot in the morning before breakfast and can be used in place of vinegar on salads. You can add a dash to a homemade juice for an extra probiotic boost or drizzle it over a soup. The leftover fermented beets can be used to make borscht, a traditional Russian soup that is said to give longevity to those who eat it.

Beet kvass is an ancient Eastern European home staple, traditionally made with aging rye bread. It was widely considered to be safer to drink than water, because contaminated water was transformed to a healthy drink during the fermentation process as the "good" bacteria overcame the "bad" bacteria.

As for all the ferments in this book, the fermentation time given in the recipe is only a guide. The temperature, amount of salt, type of water, size of the beets and microbes in your home will all help determine the outcome of your beet kvass.

Beet kvass creates a mild fizz as there is no added sugar in the ferment. While the lid needs to be on tight during primary and secondary fermentation, open it up every day or so to release some pressure, give it a good stir, and check how it tastes. Some fizzing and possibly leaking are normal during fermentation, so place the jar on a tray to collect any liquid.

FERMENTATION GUIDELINES

Beets

Cut the beets into ½- to ¾-inch (1 to 2 cm) pieces; don't grate them, as this will cause too much juice to bleed into the water, increasing the fermentation substantially and possibly creating beet wine! Choose organic beets if possible and don't peel them – just give them a good scrub with plain water. You actually want the goodness and yeasts inherent in the skins as part of the fermentation.

Salt

Salt is one of the most important ingredients in kvass. Don't use iodized table salt – it needs to be pure Himalayan salt, or unrefined sea salt. The salt is a catalyst to draw out the water from the beets and create an environment where the "good" bacteria proliferate and the "bad" bacteria aren't given a chance to take over. The additives that are used in iodized table salt can interfere with the fermentation process. Pure sea salt contains high levels of minerals to feed the "good" bacteria and encourage fermentation.

First fermentation vessel

Use a 1-quart (1 liter) wide-mouth glass, food-grade plastic or stainless steel container with a lid.

Covering

Kvass is an anaerobic fermentation process, so it does not require oxygen for fermentation. Keep the fermentation vessel and the bottle tightly closed.

Bottling

I recommend using a 3- to 4-cup (750 ml to 1 liter) sturdy glass bottle with a narrow neck and a tight-fitting lid. The lid needs a good seal so that the fizz stays in the bottle. A bottle with a flip-top rubber stopper is suitable. You will also need a strainer and a funnel.

Sediment

Some sediment (called "lees") may appear in both the first and second fermentation stages. This is normal and fine to drink.

HOW TO KNOW WHEN YOUR
BEET KVASS
IS READY FOR BOTTLING

SMELL

The kvass should have a slight lemony smell, due to the sourness of the fermentation. You should notice a change from sweet beets to a more sour liquid. There is a clearness and freshness to the smell, like freshly dug soil.

LOOK

You may see small bubbles on the side of the fermentation vessel. You should also see the liquid absorb the color of the beets, turning it the color of blood. If the liquid is quite viscous, it may have been overfermented and probably won't be pleasant to drink. It shouldn't have the consistency of a purée or tomato juice; it should be light, fresh and watery.

LISTEN

You are unlikely to hear active bubbling and fizzing during fermentation, although you may hear a "pop" when you open the bottle to "burp" it.

TASTE

The final taste of the beet kvass will vary. It's likely to taste like watered-down vegetable juice, a little salty and a little sour. It should also have a slight savory lemony taste. It will be earthy, fresh and refreshing; the flavor doesn't linger on the palate. If you are new to fermentation, I recommend you taste the kvass daily during primary fermentation to check its progress.

TROUBLESHOOTING

WHAT IF THE BREW TURNS MOLDY?

If you see mold growing, discard the beet kvass and start again. Even though the mold may be harmless, it's not worth risking your health by drinking it.

WHAT IF THE BREW IS TOO VISCOUS?

The kvass should taste watery and have a very subtle fizz. If it turns quite thick and viscous, and has a strange smell, discard the brew and try again. It may be bad due to a variety of factors, such as:

* not being stirred often enough
* an imbalance of yeasts and bacteria
* too much or too little salt
* chlorinated water.

WHAT IF THE BREW IS TOO SALTY?

If your beet kvass is too salty, you can dilute it with filtered water to make it more palatable.

WHAT IF THE BREW TURNS ALCOHOLIC?

Did you grate, rather than chop the beets? If the beet is grated or chopped too finely, it will release too many sugars and could turn alcoholic. Only use chopped beets; don't grate them.

WHAT IF I DON'T LIKE THE TASTE?

If this happens, you can use the kvass a little like a vinegar, and combine it with some salt, pepper, olive oil and lemon juice to turn it into a salad dressing.

WHAT IF MY KVASS ISN'T RED ENOUGH?

Over the course of a few days, you will see the color of the beet bleed into the clear water, leaving the finished kvass a blood-red color. If it's a very light pink color, the kvass is not ready. Allow it to ferment longer, stirring it frequently.

WHAT IF THERE IS A WHITE FILM ON MY KVASS?

This white film is generally harmless. Simply scrape it off the top of the kvass and allow the fermentation to continue.

RECIPES

basic beet kvass

Earthy and a little dirty, the beet is a titan of the health food world that is seriously undervalued. It's a crimson nugget packed with blood-cleansing antioxidants, minerals and vitamins. I love it! In my experience, there is no need to burp the kvass daily, as it's not a highly effervescent ferment.

Preparation time: 15 minutes **Fermentation time:** 5–8 days **Difficulty:** Easy
Shelf life: Refrigerate for up to 2 months **Makes:** About 3 cups (750 ml)

INGREDIENTS

2 medium or 1 large beet,
   skin intact
½ teaspoon pure sea salt
3 cups (750 ml) filtered water
   or spring water

PRIMARY FERMENTATION

Wash the beet and cut it into ½- to ¾-inch (1 to 2 cm) pieces. Put the beet in a 1-quart (1 liter) wide-mouth glass jar with a tight-fitting lid and add the salt. Pour in the filtered water, leaving a ¾-inch (2 cm) gap between the liquid and the lid. Stir to dissolve the salt.

Tightly seal the jar and place out of direct sunlight in a cool spot. Leave the liquid to ferment for 3 to 5 days, stirring or shaking daily. After around 3 days, taste the kvass. When it is as dark and sour as you like it, the kvass is ready to bottle.

BOTTLING

Put a funnel in the opening of a 3-cup (750 ml) glass bottle with a tight-fitting lid and put a strainer on top of the funnel. Pour the kvass into the bottle through the strainer. Discard the beet left in the strainer (see Tip).

SECONDARY FERMENTATION

Tightly seal the bottle lid and leave the bottle on the counter to build carbonation. This could take 2 to 3 days, depending on the temperature.

DRINK UP

When the kvass is as fizzy as you like (beet kvass only produces a mild fizz), store it in the fridge to slow the fermentation process, and enjoy cold.

———

TIP *Use the fermented beet in a salad or to make borscht, or roast and mash it with some ground cumin to make a probiotic dip.*

———

beautifying blueberry beet kvass

The fermentation process naturally enhances the nutrient profile of a food and unlocks its nutrients, making them easier to digest. Blueberries are already a potent source of antioxidants, so fermenting only makes them more powerful. Combining the fermented blueberries with the living probiotics and cleansing properties of beet kvass makes an amazing drink.

Preparation time: 15 minutes **Fermentation time:** 5–8 days **Difficulty:** Easy
Shelf life: Refrigerate for up to 2 months **Makes:** About 1 quart (1 liter)

INGREDIENTS
1 recipe basic beet kvass
(page 130)
¼ cup (35 g) fresh blueberries
and/or 1 cup (250 ml)
blueberry juice

PRIMARY FERMENTATION
Follow the instructions for basic beet kvass.

BOTTLING
Follow the instructions for basic beet kvass, using a 1-quart (1 liter) bottle.

SECONDARY FERMENTATION
Add the blueberries and/or blueberry juice to the bottle and tightly seal the lid. Leave the bottle on the counter to build carbonation. This could take 2 to 3 days, depending on the temperature.

DRINK UP
When the kvass is as fizzy as you like (beet kvass only produces a mild fizz), store it in the fridge to slow the fermentation process, and enjoy cold.

TIPS *Some blueberry juices contain lots of added sugar. Look for one that contains pure unsweetened blueberry juice.*
If you have any leftover kvass that doesn't fit into the bottle, you can drink it right away or bottle it separately.

wintry beet kvass with orange and cloves

Cloves are a perfect match for the pungent and earthy beet. They have many medicinal benefits – they are anti-inflammatory and antifungal and can even be used to deter mold in the home. Cloves are actually the flower buds of an evergreen rain forest tree, *Sygizium aromaticum*, that is native to Indonesia. The buds start off pale in color, then turn from green to bright red at the time of picking. Taste your kvass and only add a second clove at the bottling stage if you want more aroma. They're small, but they pack a lot of punch.

Preparation time: 15 minutes **Fermentation time:** 5–8 days **Difficulty:** Easy
Shelf life: Refrigerate for up to 2 months **Makes:** About 3 cups (750 ml)

INGREDIENTS
*1 recipe basic beet kvass
    (page 130)*
1 or 2 cloves
*1 drop edible pure orange
    essential oil or 2 thin strips
    orange zest*

PRIMARY FERMENTATION
Follow the instructions for basic beet kvass, adding 1 clove and 1 strip orange zest, if using, to the jar.

BOTTLING
Follow the instructions for basic beet kvass.

SECONDARY FERMENTATION
Taste the kvass and add the remaining clove, if needed, and a drop of orange oil or the remaining orange zest to the bottle. Tightly seal the bottle lid and leave the bottle on the counter to build carbonation. This could take 2 to 3 days, depending on the temperature.

DRINK UP
When the kvass is as fizzy as you like (beet kvass only produces a mild fizz), store it in the fridge to slow the fermentation process, and enjoy cold.

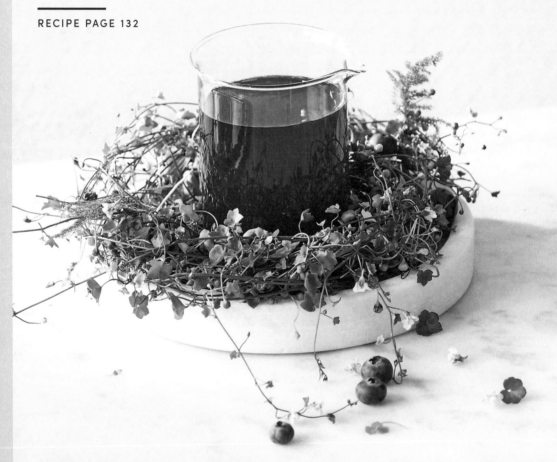

*beautifying blueberry
beet kvass*

RECIPE PAGE 132

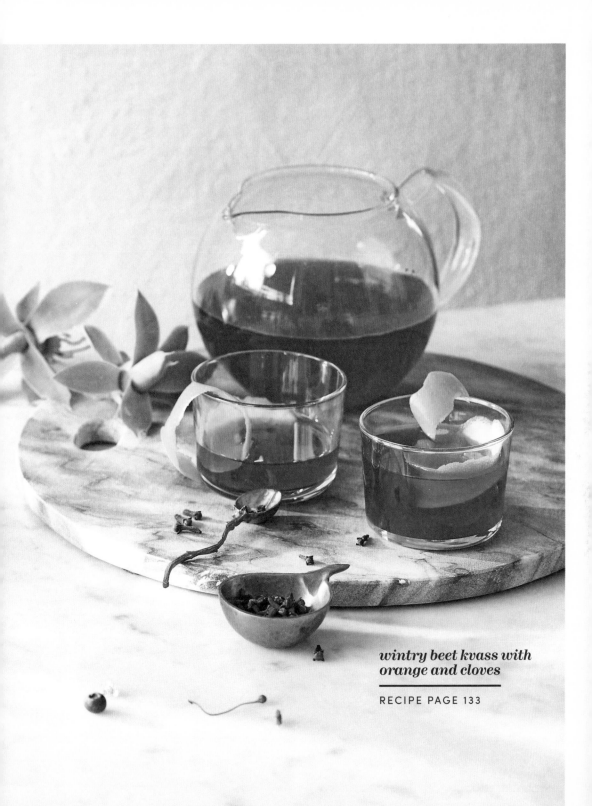

wintry beet kvass with orange and cloves

RECIPE PAGE 133

pomegranate beet kvass

Pomegranate is one of my favorite fruits. It's crimson, juicy, textural and voluptuous all at the same time, and it's been eaten since ancient times. Pomegranate contains high levels of flavonoids and polyphenols, which are potent antioxidants offering possible protection against heart disease and cancer. It's beautifully tart and lends itself perfectly to beet kvass, adding a dimension of sweetness and tartness. Use pomegranate arils (seeds), juice or a combination of the two.

Preparation time: 15 minutes **Fermentation time:** 5–8 days **Difficulty:** Easy
Shelf life: Refrigerate for up to 2 months **Makes:** About 1 quart (1 liter)

INGREDIENTS
1 recipe basic beet kvass
  (page 130)
arils (seeds) of ½ pomegranate
  or 1 cup (250 ml)
  pomegranate juice

PRIMARY FERMENTATION
Follow the instructions for basic beet kvass.

BOTTLING
Follow the instructions for basic beet kvass, using a 1-quart (1 liter) bottle.

SECONDARY FERMENTATION
Add the pomegranate arils or pomegranate juice to the bottle and tightly seal the lid. Leave the bottle on the counter to build carbonation. This could take 2 to 3 days, depending on the temperature.

DRINK UP
When the kvass is as fizzy as you like (beet kvass only produces a mild fizz), store it in the fridge to slow the fermentation process, and enjoy cold.

TIP *If you have any leftover kvass that doesn't fit into the bottle, you can drink it right away or bottle it separately.*

beet kvass with blood orange

I'm really drawn to blood oranges. There's something rich and beautiful about the way the colors bleed and swirl into each other. Blood oranges are high in vitamin C and contain anthocyanin, a pigment and antioxidant that gives blood oranges their crimson color. When you combine the probiotic power and living enzymes in the beet kvass with the antioxidants from the blood orange, you end up with a superpowerful drink.

Preparation time: 15 minutes **Fermentation time:** 5–8 days **Difficulty:** Easy
Shelf life: Refrigerate for up to 2 months **Makes:** About 3 cups (750 ml)

INGREDIENTS
1 recipe basic beet kvass
(page 130)
1 strip blood orange zest
juice of 1 blood orange

PRIMARY FERMENTATION
Follow the instructions for basic beet kvass.

BOTTLING
Follow the instructions for basic beet kvass.

SECONDARY FERMENTATION
Add the orange zest and juice to the bottle and tightly seal the lid. Leave the bottle on the counter to build carbonation. This could take 2 to 3 days, depending on the temperature.

DRINK UP
When the kvass is as fizzy as you like (beet kvass only produces a mild fizz), store it in the fridge to slow the fermentation process, and enjoy cold.

TIP *If blood oranges aren't available, use any citrus you enjoy.*

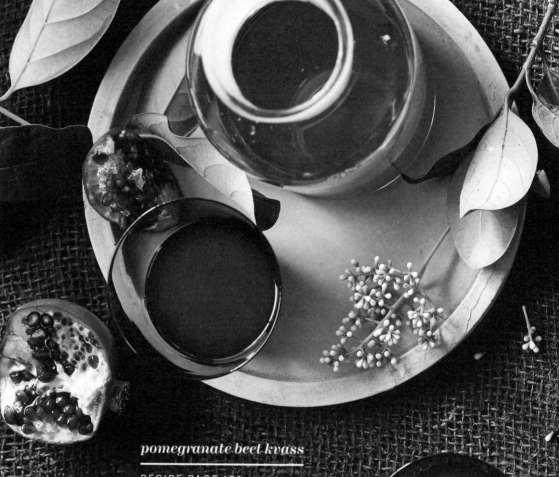

pomegranate beet kvass

RECIPE PAGE 136

beet kvass with blood orange

RECIPE PAGE 137

roots and rhizomes kvass

RECIPE PAGE 140

roots and rhizomes kvass

With its incredibly vibrant color, turmeric is one of my all-time favorite spices. It's high in curcumin, which is anti-inflammatory, as well as antioxidants, and the nutrient profile increases when you ferment it. Ginger is another fabulous spice, long esteemed for its digestion-enhancing properties and the ability to relieve nausea. When you sip this medicinal beet kvass, you will be reaping the benefits of these gorgeous spices, as well as enhancing your microbiome with living probiotics.

Preparation time: 15 minutes **Fermentation time:** 5–8 days **Difficulty:** Easy
Shelf life: Refrigerate for up to 2 months **Makes:** About 1 quart (1 liter)

INGREDIENTS
1 recipe basic beet kvass
  (page 130)
1 sliver fresh turmeric
1 sliver fresh ginger
freshly cracked black pepper
  (optional)

PRIMARY FERMENTATION
Follow the instructions for basic beet kvass, adding the turmeric and ginger to the jar before you seal it.

BOTTLING
Follow the instructions for basic beet kvass, reserving the fermented turmeric and ginger.

SECONDARY FERMENTATION
Add the reserved turmeric, ginger and a pinch of black pepper, if using, to the bottle. Tightly seal the bottle lid and leave the bottle on the counter to build carbonation. This could take 2 to 3 days, depending on the temperature.

DRINK UP
When the kvass is as fizzy as you like (beet kvass only produces a mild fizz), store it in the fridge to slow the fermentation process, and enjoy cold.

TIPS *The black pepper will increase the body's absorption of the turmeric.*
  Use the fermented ginger and turmeric slivers in your morning juice or in a stir-fry.

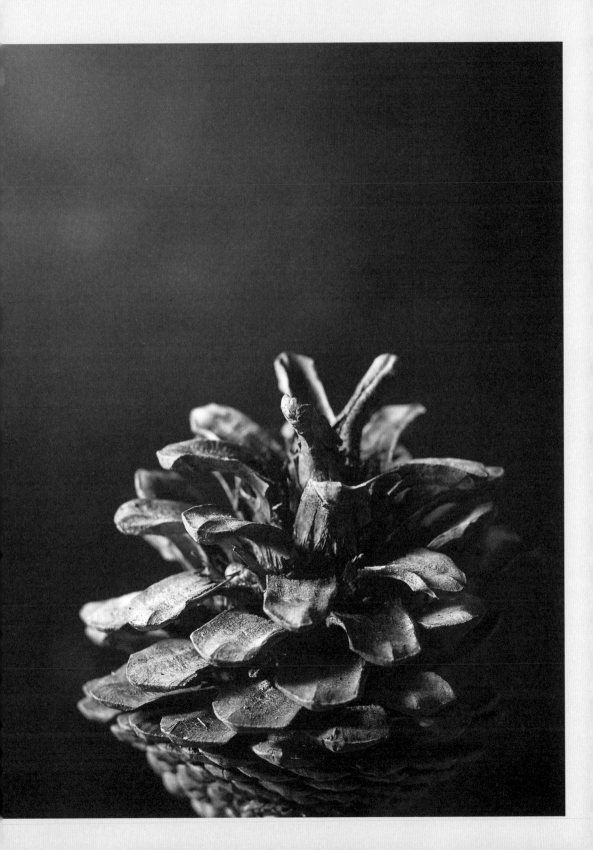

6. PINEAPPLE TEPACHE

Everything about pineapple tepache screams, "Summer!"
It's a sweet, fizzy and absolutely delightful probiotic drink that's simple
to make, utterly affordable and uses pineapple skin scraps: sustainability
in action. This is wild fermentation at its best.

Pineapple tepache originated with the Nahua people in pre-Columbian Mexico. The word *tepache* translates as "drink made from corn." This is how the drink was originally fermented.

When my husband and I were backpacking around Mexico we often purchased pineapple tepache from one of the many street vendors or market stalls. The tepache was sold in a plastic bag, which was sealed at the top using a rubber band and had a straw poked into the side. The taste of the sweet and bubbly pineapple-flavored liquid instantly transports me back to that time in my life when things were easy and breezy.

The fermentation process for pineapple tepache is simple, quick and easy to master. It relies on the wild yeasts that live on the pineapple skin and in the environment to convert the sugars. I have tried making tepache using pineapple flesh rather than the skin but the result was a less vigorous, less fermented brew.

Essentially, you can adapt the essence of this recipe to make any fruit-infused probiotic drink you like. Keep the sugar and water ratios the same, but replace the pineapple skins with apple skins, raspberries, strawberries or any other fruit that's in season.

FERMENTATION GUIDELINES

Pineapple

Choose organic pineapple if possible.

Sugar

Raw sugar or light brown sugar can be used in pineapple tepache. If you use light brown sugar, the tepache will have a slight molasses taste, whereas using raw sugar will result in a lighter flavor.

First fermentation vessel

Use a heatproof 2-quart (2 liter) wide-mouth glass, food-grade plastic or stainless steel container.

Covering

Tepache is an aerobic fermentation process, so it likes oxygen in the first fermentation stage. Cover the fermentation vessel with a piece of cheesecloth or clean dry dusting cloth and secure it with a rubber band.

During the secondary fermentation, the bottle needs to be tightly sealed with a lid to allow the carbonation to develop.

Bottling

I recommend using two 1-quart (1 liter) sturdy glass bottles with narrow necks and tight-fitting lids (similar to champagne bottles) as this shape will encourage carbonation to develop. The lids need a good seal so that the fizz stays in the bottles. Bottles with flip-top rubber stoppers are suitable. You will also need a strainer and a funnel.

Sediment

Some sediment (called "lees") may appear in both the first and second fermentation stages. This is normal. Either stir it up and add it to your finished tepache or discard it.

HOW TO KNOW WHEN YOUR
— *PINEAPPLE TEPACHE* —
IS READY FOR BOTTLING

SMELL

The tepache should have a slight vinegary smell – the smell of sweet pineapple will be present, but it will be a little more acidic.

LOOK

You should see small bubbles on the side of the fermentation vessel. There may be some white foam on top of the pineapple skins, and you may see bubbles rising up from the bottom of the jar to the top. This is fermentation in action.

LISTEN

You may be able to hear the fermentation ticking along with the sound of fizzing and hissing.

TASTE

You should notice a change in flavor from sweet to a little more savory as the fermentation develops. The finished tepache tastes almost buttery, with toasted caramel flavors. It has a delicate balance between sweet and savory. It's light on the palate and very clean and refreshing.

TROUBLESHOOTING

WHAT IF THE BREW TURNS MOLDY?

If you see mold growing, discard the tepache and start again. Even though the mold may be harmless, it's not worth risking your health.

WHAT IF THE BREW ISN'T FERMENTING?

If your tepache is not fermenting after 7 days, ask yourself the following questions:

Have you been regularly and vigorously stirring the tepache?

Is the brew too cold? Try moving it to a warmer spot to ferment.

Does it have enough sugar?

Are there pesticides on the pineapple skins? These could inhibit fermentation.

WHAT IF THE BREW IS TOO THICK?

If your tepache is quite thick and viscous, it's generally still fine to drink – it just may be sweeter than you would like it. You can use it like a cordial and dilute it with sparkling mineral water or soda water.

WHAT IF THERE IS A WHITE FILM ON MY TEPACHE?

This cloudy white film or foam is generally harmless. Simply scoop it off before bottling or when you see it develop.

WHAT IF MY TEPACHE ISN'T SWEET ENOUGH?

If you prefer your drinks on the sweeter side, add more sugar at the first fermentation stage and the resulting drink will be sweeter.

WHAT IF MY TEPACHE HAS FERMENTED FOR TOO LONG AND TURNED INTO VINEGAR?

Lucky you! This is the later stage of fermentation, when the bacteria and yeasts have consumed all the sugars from the pineapple and sugar water, leaving you with a pineapple vinegar. Use this as a gut-tonic shot, or mix it with olive oil to make a salad dressing.

WHAT IF MY TEPACHE ISN'T FIZZY ENOUGH?

Once the tepache has been bottled, you need to leave it long enough for it to develop carbonation. This could take up to a week in cold temperatures and as little as 12 hours in hotter temperatures.

WHAT IF THE TEPACHE TURNS ALCOHOLIC?

All ferments are naturally a little alcoholic, but the high sugar content of pineapple means that tepache has the potential to become more alcoholic than other ferments. Enjoy it cold at happy hour on a hot night, or as a spritzer mixed with some sparkling mineral water or coconut water.

RECIPES

basic pineapple tepache

This sweet, bubbly and fragrant drink is supremely hydrating and evokes the feeling of being on a tropical island with the sun on your back and the salt in your hair. Try to catch the ferment just in time – the longer it ferments, the more alcohol it will produce and it could turn vinegary and a little viscous.

Preparation time: 15 minutes **Fermentation time:** 2–10 days **Difficulty:** Easy
Shelf life: Refrigerate for up to 2 months **Makes:** About 2 quarts (2 liters)

INGREDIENTS

2 quarts (2 liters) filtered water or spring water
1 cup (220 g) raw sugar or 1 cup (185 g) lightly packed light brown sugar
1 pineapple

PRIMARY FERMENTATION

Bring 1 cup (250 ml) of the filtered water to the boil. Add the sugar to a heatproof 2-quart (2 liter) wide-mouth glass jar. Pour in the boiling water and stir well to dissolve the sugar. Add enough of the remaining filtered water to three-quarters fill the jar and set aside to cool.

Wash the outside of the pineapple. Using a sharp knife, cut off the pineapple skin, leaving a little flesh attached. Add the pineapple skins to the sugar-water solution and stir vigorously. Top up with filtered water to fill the jar, if necessary, then stir again. Cover the jar with a piece of cheesecloth and secure with a rubber band.

Place the jar out of direct sunlight in a warm spot and leave to ferment for 1 to 7 days, depending on the temperature. If it's very hot, check after 12 hours as that may be sufficient time for fermentation to take effect. Give the tepache a vigorous stir each day and check the taste. If the pineapple skins have popped out of the liquid, push them back down to reduce the chance of the tepache becoming moldy.

BOTTLING

Remove and discard the pineapple skins and skim off any foam and scum from the top of the tepache.

Put a funnel in the opening of a 1-quart (1 liter) glass bottle with a tight-fitting lid and put a strainer on top of the funnel. Pour half the tepache into the bottle through the strainer. Repeat with a second 1-quart (1 liter) bottle and the remaining tepache.

SECONDARY FERMENTATION

Tightly seal the bottle lids and leave the bottles on the counter to build carbonation. This could take 1 to 3 days, depending on the temperature. "Burp" the tepache daily to release some pressure by opening the lids slightly and then tightening them again. Depending on the residual sugars and the fermentation activity, pressure can build significantly. In order to prevent an explosion, test the fizz every couple of days.

DRINK UP

When the tepache is as fizzy as you like (this could range from a small spritz to a ferocious fizz), store it in the fridge to slow the fermentation process, and enjoy cold.

——

TIP *For a truly delicious and grown-up drink, use the pineapple tepache in place of pineapple juice in your next piña colada.*

——

mint pineapple tepache

The addition of mint is pretty and adds a freshness and crispness to the tepache. It's a cooling and soothing herb that helps ease digestion and tummy troubles, and a perfect choice for summer because of the cooling effect it has on the body.

Preparation time: 15 minutes **Fermentation time:** 2–10 days **Difficulty:** Easy
Shelf life: Refrigerate for up to 2 months **Makes:** About 2 quarts (2 liters)

INGREDIENTS

1 recipe basic pineapple tepache (page 146)
2 mint sprigs

PRIMARY FERMENTATION

Follow the instructions for basic pineapple tepache.

BOTTLING

Follow the instructions for basic pineapple tepache.

SECONDARY FERMENTATION

Add a mint sprig to each bottle and tightly seal the lids. Leave the bottles on the counter to build carbonation. This could take 1 to 3 days, depending on the temperature. "Burp" the tepache daily to release some pressure by opening the lids slightly and then tightening them again. Depending on the residual sugars and the fermentation activity, pressure can build significantly. In order to prevent an explosion, test the fizz every couple of days.

DRINK UP

When the tepache is as fizzy as you like (this could range from a small spritz to a ferocious fizz), store it in the fridge to slow the fermentation process, and enjoy cold.

TIP *Serve this tepache over ice cubes made from coconut water for a tropical treat.*

Mexican pineapple tepache with cinnamon

This variation is a classic in Mexico. The beautiful digestive qualities of the probiotic tepache are coupled with the botanical properties of the cinnamon. The cinnamon also adds a depth and warmth to the sweet pineapple and enhances the flavor of the tepache. You can use the cinnamon stick as a straw to drink your tepache.

Preparation time: 15 minutes **Fermentation time:** 2–10 days **Difficulty:** Easy
Shelf life: Refrigerate for up to 2 months **Makes:** About 2 quarts (2 liters)

INGREDIENTS
*1 recipe basic pineapple tepache
    (page 146)*
2 cinnamon sticks

PRIMARY FERMENTATION
Follow the instructions for basic pineapple tepache.

BOTTLING
Follow the instructions for basic pineapple tepache.

SECONDARY FERMENTATION
Add a cinnamon stick to each bottle and tightly seal the lids. Leave the bottles on the counter to build carbonation. This could take 1 to 3 days, depending on the temperature. "Burp" the tepache daily to release some pressure by opening the lids slightly and then tightening them again. Depending on the residual sugars and the fermentation activity, pressure can build significantly. In order to prevent an explosion, test the fizz every couple of days.

DRINK UP
When the tepache is as fizzy as you like (this could range from a small spritz to a ferocious fizz), store it in the fridge to slow the fermentation process, and enjoy cold.

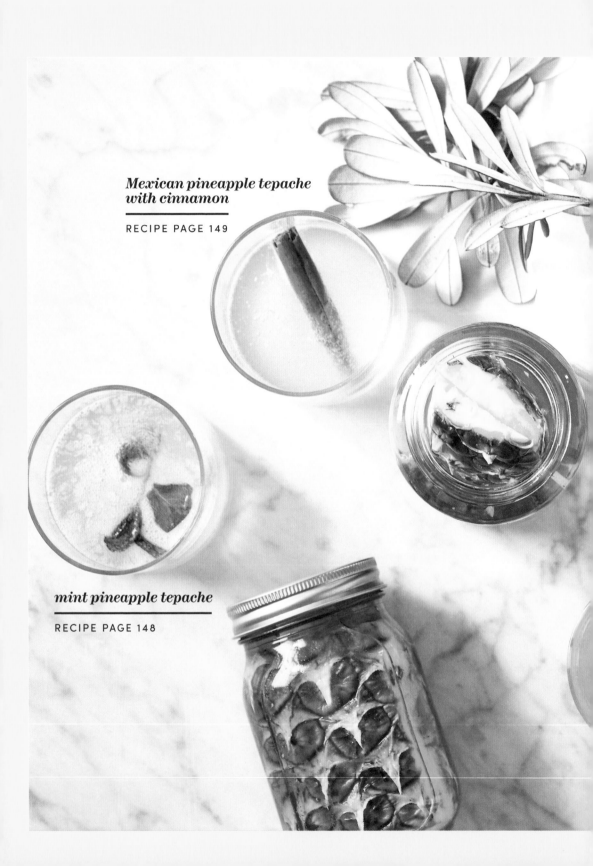

**Mexican pineapple tepache
with cinnamon**

RECIPE PAGE 149

mint pineapple tepache

RECIPE PAGE 148

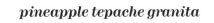

pineapple tepache granita

RECIPE PAGE 153

chile pineapple tepache

RECIPE PAGE 152

chile pineapple tepache

This is my favorite tepache recipe. The fire and depth of the chile marries delightfully with the intense sweetness and fragrance of the tepache. Chiles can contain up to seven times the vitamin C of oranges, are rich in antioxidants and can heat up digestive fires. Chiles have different potencies, with the seeds packing more punch than the flesh, so adjust according to your preference. I like to split the chile down the center before I add it to the bottle. You could substitute cayenne pepper for fresh chile.

Preparation time: 15 minutes **Fermentation time:** 2–10 days **Difficulty:** Easy
Shelf life: Refrigerate for up to 2 months **Makes:** About 2 quarts (2 liters)

INGREDIENTS
1 recipe basic pineapple tepache
(page 146)
1 fresh long red chile, cut in half
lengthwise, or 2 fresh small
red chiles

PRIMARY FERMENTATION
Follow the instructions for basic pineapple tepache.

BOTTLING
Follow the instructions for basic pineapple tepache.

SECONDARY FERMENTATION
Add half the chile to each bottle and tightly seal the lids. Leave the bottles on the counter to build carbonation. This could take 1 to 3 days, depending on the temperature. "Burp" the tepache daily to release some pressure by opening the lids slightly and then tightening them again. Depending on the residual sugars and the fermentation activity, pressure can build significantly. In order to prevent an explosion, test the fizz every couple of days.

DRINK UP
When the tepache is as fizzy as you like (this could range from a small spritz to a ferocious fizz), store it in the fridge to slow the fermentation process, and enjoy cold.

pineapple tepache granita

Granita is a semifrozen dish that has its origins in Sicily. The texture can vary from coarse and icy to smooth and sorbet-like. This is a chunky-style granita with large ice crystals. It makes a lovely palate cleanser between courses over a long summer lunch. For a granita with a smoother, sorbet-like texture, whisk in 2 egg whites just before freezing. Freeze until completely firm, then cut the mixture into cubes and process in a high-speed blender until silky smooth.

Preparation time: 15 minutes **Freezing time:** 2–3 hours **Difficulty:** Medium
Shelf life: Freeze for up to 2 months **Makes:** About 2 quarts (2 liters)

INGREDIENTS
*1 recipe basic pineapple tepache
    (page 146)*
*mint sprigs or pomegranate arils
    (seeds), to serve (optional)*

FREEZING
Pour the bottled tepache into a 10-cup (2.5 liter) shallow tray.
    Freeze the mixture, uncovered, for 2 to 3 hours. If you have the time, you can scrape a fork or spoon through the mixture every 30 minutes to make ice granules. Alternatively, leave it in the freezer to set completely, then scrape a large, heavy spoon across the surface to make shaved ice.

EAT UP
Scoop the granita into chilled glasses and garnish with mint sprigs or pomegranate arils, if using.

7. GINGER BUG

Ginger bug is the bubbly, yeasty and lively liquid that is created when fresh ginger, sugar and water are left to naturally ferment with the aid of wild yeasts in the air. You don't drink the ginger bug on its own – it's the starter culture from which you make ginger beer and a variety of other beers.

A ginger bug is easy and inexpensive to start up. Given the right care and environment, it will stay alive and bubbling for a lifetime and continue to nourish you for many years with its probiotic goodness – I'm planning on handing down some living cultures to my children as heirlooms. Think of the ginger bug as a friend who only needs to be fed and stirred daily in return for taking care of your gut health.

When you make a ginger bug, you invite the wild yeasts and good bacteria that live in your home and the air to come and lend a hand. It's amazing that a simple combination of fresh air, time, water, sugar and ginger can create such wonderful results.

Once stage one is complete and the ginger bug is ready, it's time to move on to stage two and make the ginger beer. This involves taking out a little of the ginger bug and adding it to another mixture of ginger, water and sugar, then bottling it and leaving it to become fizzy. You will need to leave about half of the ginger bug behind so that you have a starter culture ready for next time. Don't be concerned about the amount of sugar you add to these recipes. The sugar is there to attract the wild yeasts to activate the wild fermentation process. The

yeasts eat up most of the sugar, leaving a low-sugar drink. This probiotic-rich, effervescent and classic ginger beer is one of the best things to happen to ginger and your tummy.

It's such a shame that we have, for the most part, forgotten these home-fermenting skills and missed out on the fun of watching life spring forth from staple ingredients. Here's your chance to reintroduce this family tradition. Once you've mastered the basics, you can go ahead and experiment with new flavors.

A WORD ABOUT GINGER

When making a ginger bug, you need to leave the skin on the ginger as it contains a lot of the yeasts that are put to work in this fermentation. Most supermarket-bought ginger has been sprayed to help prolong its shelf life. This spray could interfere with the fermentation process, so I recommend using organic ginger. However, I have made ginger bug using nonorganic ginger and it worked, so if you don't have access to organic ginger, you can give it a try. If it doesn't work it may be because the good bacteria and yeasts can't proliferate.

FERMENTATION GUIDELINES

Ginger

You need a large piece of ginger, about the size of your hand. This is chopped and added to the fermenting ginger bug over the course of a week or so. Leave the skin on the ginger.

Sugar

You can use white, raw or light brown sugar for the ginger bug. There are more minerals in raw or light brown sugar, which the ginger bug prefers, but most sugars tend to work.

Fermentation vessel

Use a 2-cup (500 ml) wide-mouth glass, food-grade plastic or stainless-steel container or drinking glass to ferment the ginger bug. As it grows, you can gradually increase the size of the fermentation vessel.

Covering

Ginger bug is an aerobic fermentation process, so it likes access to oxygen to keep fermentation happening. Cover the fermentation vessel with a piece of cheesecloth or clean dry dusting cloth and secure it with a rubber band.

Feeding

The ginger bug is alive and needs to be fed and stirred often. Choose from the following two feeding options.

1. Leave the ginger bug in the container on the kitchen counter and feed it 1 teaspoon of chopped ginger and 1 teaspoon of white, raw or light brown sugar a couple of times a week. Stir it as often as you can, at least every 2 days but preferably daily.

2. Put the ginger bug in the fridge. Once a week, feed it 1 teaspoon of chopped ginger and 1 teaspoon of white, raw or light brown sugar. When you're ready to use it, add 1 tablespoon plus 1 teaspoon of sugar and 1 tablespoon plus 1 teaspoon of ginger to reactivate it and stir vigorously.

Taking a break from fermenting

The ginger bug should be fine if it's immersed in a sugar-water solution (see below) and then refrigerated for up to 6 weeks. It may need a couple of weeks of feeding and stirring before it's bubbling again, so be patient.

RESTING THE GINGER BUG

If you go away or want to take a break from fermenting, you need to rest the ginger bug in the fridge to slow down fermentation.

SUGAR-WATER SOLUTION

1 cup (220 g) raw sugar
2 cups (500 ml) filtered water
*   or spring water*

Put the sugar in a glass or food-grade plastic container. Add the filtered water and stir to dissolve the sugar.

Add the ginger bug to the container. Cover the container with cheesecloth, a plate or a very loose-fitting lid and store in the fridge for up to 6 weeks.

HOW TO KNOW WHEN YOUR
GINGER BUG ——
IS READY TO MAKE GINGER BEER AND ROOT BEER

SMELL

The ginger bug should have a slightly sour and yeasty smell – you will notice the change from sweet sugar water to sour and a little sharp. You should be able to smell a distinctive brewery or yeasty smell.

LOOK

You will notice the active fermentation happening – there should be bubbles forming. It's amazing to watch!

LISTEN

There could be a soft, audible bubbling sound as the ginger bug ferments.

TASTE OF THE BOTTLED GINGER BEER OR ROOT BEER

The taste will change from sweet sugar water to tangy, a little sharp and a little sour. There should be some bubbles on your tongue.

TROUBLESHOOTING

WHAT IF THE GINGER BUG TURNS MOLDY?

Occasionally (but unusually), mold can develop on the ginger bug. Discard this bug and start again – it's not worth risking your health.

WHAT IF THE GINGER BUG DOESN'T SEEM TO BE BUBBLING?

A healthy ginger bug should start to visibly bubble. It could take up to 10 days before this happens. If the bug doesn't seem to be bubbling after 10 days, ask yourself the following:

Is your water chlorinated? Use filtered water or spring water.

Is your sugar too refined? Use raw sugar or light brown sugar.

Is it too cold? The ginger bug prefers to ferment between 68°F (20°C) and 86°F (30°C).

Are there preservatives on your ginger? Make sure you use organic ginger as any chemicals can kill the delicate balance of yeasts and bacteria.

Are you stirring and feeding the ginger bug daily?

WHAT IF MY BEER DOESN'T BECOME FIZZY?

Generally, ginger beer and root beer produce an incredible amount of fizz, as the bacteria and yeasts love the ginger. If, however, your ginger or root beer is not fizzing after the secondary fermentation, it's probably because the ginger bug was not active enough. Check that the ginger bug is bubbly when you add it, that there is no soap residue on any of the fermentation vessels and there is sufficient sugar. A healthy ginger bug will produce a healthy beer, so get the ginger bug right and the rest should follow.

RECIPES

ginger bug

A ginger bug is the base culture you can use to make a variety of other probiotic fizzy drinks. The bug is self-perpetuating – that is, start it off right, get it bubbling and it should continue to ferment, ready and waiting for you to make your next probiotic drink. Once the ginger bug has "taken" and is bubbling away (this usually takes 3 to 10 days), it's ready to make into your chosen drink. The ginger bug is only active when it's bubbling, so the key to successfully fermenting ginger beer and root beer is to use an actively bubbling ginger bug.

Preparation time: 15 minutes **Fermentation time:** 3–10 days **Difficulty:** Hard
Shelf life: Indefinite (with correct care) **Makes:** 2 cups (500 ml)

INGREDIENTS

1 large piece fresh ginger, about the size of your hand, finely chopped

1 cup (185 g) lightly packed light brown sugar or 1 cup (220 g) white sugar

1 cup (250 ml) filtered water or spring water

PRIMARY FERMENTATION

Add ¼ cup (25 g) of the finely chopped ginger to a 2-cup (500 ml) wide-mouth glass jar.

Add ¼ cup (45 g) of the sugar to the jar, then pour the filtered water over the mixture. Stir well to combine and dissolve the sugar.

Cover the jar with a piece of cheesecloth and secure with a rubber band. Place the jar out of direct sunlight in a warm spot and leave to ferment.

Once a day, add 1 tablespoon plus 1 teaspoon of the chopped ginger and 1 tablespoon plus 1 teaspoon of the sugar to the ginger bug and stir well. Re-cover and leave in a warm spot to ferment. Continue this process every day until the ginger bug starts to bubble. It is then ready to use to make ginger beer or root beer.

Whenever you use the ginger bug, retain half of the liquid in the fermentation jar, ready for your next brew. Follow the feeding guidelines on page 155 to keep the ginger bug alive.

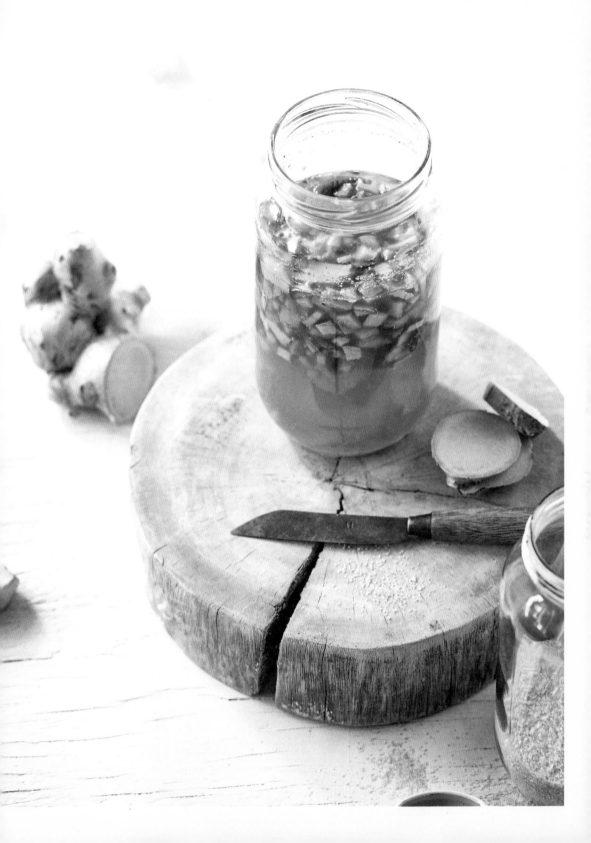

ginger beer

Who can remember the hazy taste of Grandpa's ginger beer, left in milk crates under the house while the fizz built up? My mum remembers the sound of exploding bottles left for too long over summer and the resulting sticky cleanup. This is the classic ginger beer prepared the traditional way using a ginger bug. It's full of living probiotics and digestive enzymes and is very settling for the tummy. Serve it with a squeeze of lemon or lime juice on a hot day.

Preparation time: 30 minutes **Fermentation time:** 12–72 hours **Difficulty:** Medium
Shelf life: Refrigerate for up to 4 weeks **Makes:** About 1 quart (1 liter)

INGREDIENTS

*1 large handful grated fresh
    ginger, or to taste*
*1 quart (1 liter) filtered water or
    spring water*
*¼ cup (55 g) white sugar or
    raw sugar*
*½ cup (125 ml) ginger bug
    (page 158)*

PREPARATION

Put the grated ginger and 2 cups (500 ml) of the filtered water in a saucepan. Cover and simmer for about 15 minutes. The remaining liquid should have a potent ginger flavor. Add the sugar and stir to dissolve.

When the liquid has cooled to room temperature, pour in the ginger bug and add enough of the remaining filtered water to make up 1 quart (1 liter). Stir well.

BOTTLING

Put a funnel in the opening of a 1-quart (1 liter) sturdy glass bottle with a narrow neck and a tight-fitting lid (similar to a champagne bottle). Slowly pour the ginger beer into the bottle.

FERMENTATION

Tightly seal the bottle lid and leave the bottle on the counter to build carbonation. This could take anywhere from 12 to 72 hours, depending on the temperature. The ginger beer could create forceful carbonation. In order to prevent an explosion, "burp" it daily to release some pressure by opening the lid slightly and then tightening it again.

DRINK UP

When the ginger beer is as fizzy as you like, store it in the fridge to slow the fermentation process, and enjoy cold.

———

TIPS *I like to include the grated ginger when bottling because I like spicy ginger beer. If you prefer a lighter ginger flavor, pour the ginger beer into the bottle through a strainer and discard the ginger before bottling.*

This drink will keep for 4 weeks in the fridge. Be aware that the longer it's left out of the fridge, the more fizzy it will become and there will be more risk of the bottle exploding.

———

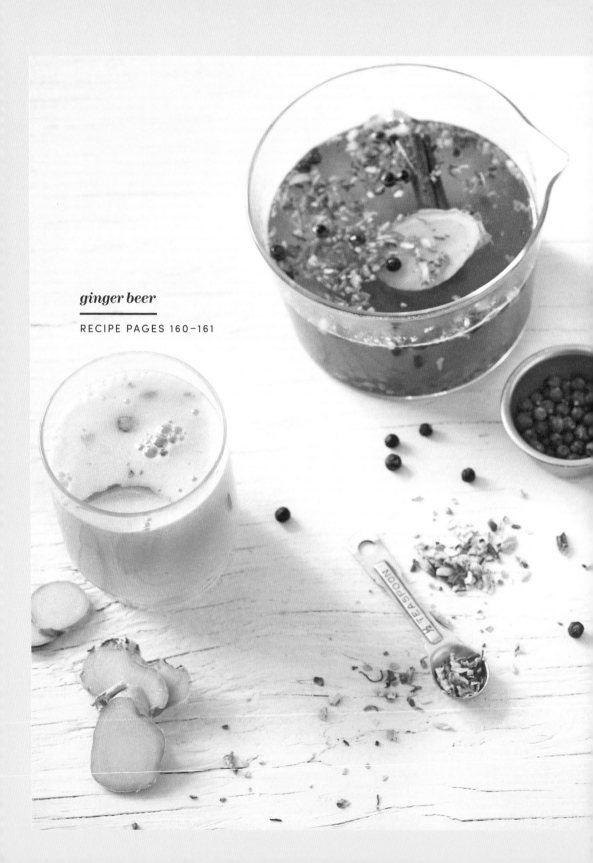

ginger beer

RECIPE PAGES 160–161

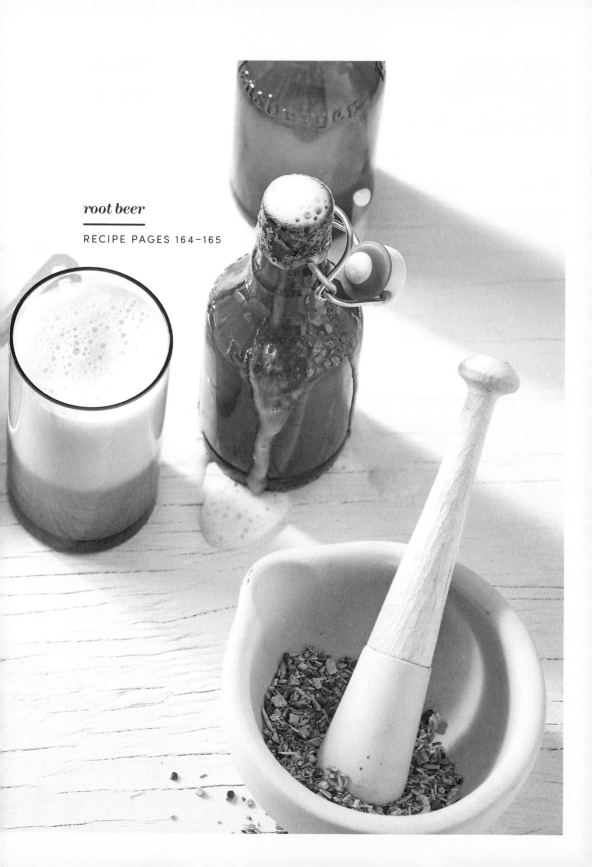

root beer

RECIPE PAGES 164–165

root beer

Root beer was one of my favorite drinks when I was growing up. Instead of the excessive sugar and artificial ingredients of commercial root beer, this beautifully healthy and vibrant version uses traditional medicinal roots, including sarsaparilla, licorice and juniper berry. There is something so charming and old-worldly about boiling down roots, barks and berries to make a fizzy drink. If you don't have access to these particular ingredients, just use what you have – any type of herb or spice will do. Try aniseed, star anise, clove or cardamom. You could even create your own blend and give the to friends as a beautiful and unique gift.

Preparation time: 15 minutes **Fermentation time:** 12–72 hours **Difficulty:** Hard
Shelf life: Refrigerate for up to 4 weeks **Makes:** About 1 quart (1 liter)

INGREDIENTS

1 teaspoon finely chopped
    sarsaparilla root
1 teaspoon finely chopped
    fresh ginger
1 teaspoon finely chopped
    licorice root
½ teaspoon finely chopped
    birch bark
1 juniper berry
1 cinnamon stick
1 quart (1 liter) filtered water or
    spring water
¼ cup (55 g) white sugar
½ cup (125 ml) ginger bug
    (page 158)

PREPARATION

Put the roots, herbs, spices, and 2 cups (500 ml) of the filtered water in a saucepan. Cover and simmer for about 15 minutes. The remaining liquid should have a potent medicinal herb flavor. Add the sugar and stir to dissolve.

When the liquid has cooled to room temperature, pour in the ginger bug and add enough of the remaining filtered water to make up 1 quart (1 liter). Stir well.

BOTTLING

Put a funnel in the opening of a 1-quart (1 liter) sturdy glass bottle with a narrow neck and a tight-fitting lid (similar to a champagne bottle). Put a strainer on top of the funnel. Pour the root beer into the bottle through the strainer. Discard the solids left in the strainer.

FERMENTATION

Tightly seal the bottle lid and leave the bottle on the counter to build carbonation. This could take anywhere from 12 to 72 hours, depending on the temperature. The root beer could create forceful carbonation. In order to prevent an explosion, "burp" it daily to release some pressure by opening the lid slightly and then tightening it again.

DRINK UP

When the root beer is as fizzy as you like, store it in the fridge to slow the fermentation process, and enjoy cold.

8. HONEY MEAD

I love honey mead. It's known as "the drink of love" and "nectar from the gods."
According to legend, after a bride and groom said their wedding vows in centuries
past, they'd be sent to the bedchamber with a bottle of sultry honey mead
to set the mood.

Honey mead is generally regarded as the ancestor of fermented drinks as it's reported to be the oldest known alcoholic beverage. An elaborate tomb containing a male body was discovered in an archaeological site in Turkey in 1957. The tomb dates back to around 740 BCE and contained 157 bronze vessels that were presumably used during a farewell burial toast. When archaeologists analyzed residues inside the vessels, they found evidence that honey mead was one of the drinks used in this ancient toast.

Time is a great asset in fermentation and honey mead is unique in that it can ferment for years before you drink it. It's a joy to open up a bottle that's been patiently fermenting for over a year. During this long, slow fermentation period, the naturally occurring bacteria and yeasts that live in the air and on surfaces we touch convert the sugars and other nutrients into a nutritious elixir that is literally bubbling with goodness.

There are various opinions about how long honey mead should be left to ferment. I've had very young honey mead that has only fermented for 1 week in summer and enjoyed it immensely, and I've also left it to ferment for up to a year. When you are just beginning your fermentation journey, I recommend that you drink your mead young – that is, after between 1 and 8 weeks of fermentation. Consider this a suggestion and allow your senses, lifestyle and instinct to guide you.

Be aware that honey mead is indeed an alcoholic elixir – my home alcohol tests show that the alcohol level is around 5 percent after 4 weeks of fermentation. The process of fermenting sugars (in this case, honey) into alcohol is spontaneous and does not require human intervention. Even overripe fruit can turn alcoholic.

The range of herbs and spices used to flavor mead can determine its classification.

* "Traditional" mead is made with only honey, water and wild yeasts.
* "Metheglin" is mead made with added herbs or spices, such as cloves or cinnamon. The word *metheglin* is an English transliteration of the Welsh word *meddyglyn*, which means "medicine."
* "Melomel" is traditional mead that has fruit added to it.
* "Rhodomel" is mead that has rose petals added to it.

CHOOSING THE HONEY

The type of honey you use in the honey mead will affect the final product. I prefer to use a light and subtle honey as this lets the spices you add come through on the palate, but you may choose to use a dark, richer honey such as buckwheat. You will find a variety of different types of honey at your local farmers' market or health food store. Try a selection of different varieties and see which one you fall in love with.

If there is any crystallization in the honey, this is a good sign because it means the honey is raw or unpasteurized and therefore supports a healthier culture of bacteria and yeasts during the fermentation process. I don't advise using creamed honey as it's been processed and will be harder to manipulate.

It's interesting to note that raw honey always has the potential to ferment when it's diluted with water because it naturally contains plenty of yeasts that can kickstart fermentation.

SPARKLING OR STILL?

The fizziness of your honey mead will ultimately be affected by how much sugar is left in the liquid after fermentation, as well as the types of yeasts that are naturally present in your home environment.

If you bottle your honey mead "young" (after a week or so of fermentation), there will be a lot of sugars in it that will convert to carbon dioxide. This will probably make more fizz and the mead will be more alcoholic.

Please be aware that this extra sugar will mean the honey mead continues to ferment in the bottle and could explode. In order to prevent an explosion, "burp" the mead every couple of days to release some pressure by opening the lid slightly and then tightening it again. When you start to see lots of fizz building up, it's best to refrigerate the mead to slow down fermentation.

If you prefer your honey mead fizzier, add about a tablespoon of honey when bottling the mead. The yeasts will convert these extra sugars and leave you with a decidedly fizzy brew. Because there is a risk of an explosion, it's important to "burp" the mead regularly.

If you prefer still honey mead, you need to let it finish its fermentation. Still mead will take much longer to ferment (as long as a year) and should not taste sweet. When you bottle it, don't add any honey as it will reactivate the yeasts. Just bottle it and store it in the fridge. Depending on a variety of factors including the nature of the honey, the temperature and the activity of the yeasts, the final product will vary from sweet to quite dry.

A NOTE ON STIRRING

Vigorous stirring aerates the liquid and helps dissolve the honey so that the wild yeasts can proliferate and ferment into honey mead. The yeasts need to have some oxygen to keep them alive, which is why opening the lid to "burp" and stir the honey mead is necessary for it to carry on fermenting.

During first fermentation, frequently take the lid off the jar and stir the honey mead with gusto to get the wild yeasts activated. Don't worry if you can't do this every day or week, as long as you get to it at some stage.

— HONEY MEAD —

FERMENTATION GUIDELINES

Honey

Choose raw unpasteurized honey if possible, as it has more living properties for the wild bacteria and yeasts to ferment. Heat-treated or pasteurized honey should work, but raw honey is the gold standard as it has more potential for fermentation.

Fermentation vessel

Use a 6-cup (1.5 liter) wide-mouth glass or food-grade plastic jar with a tight-fitting lid to ferment the honey mead. Metal is no good for honey mead (you can use metal utensils).

Covering

Mead is an anaerobic fermentation process, so it does not require oxygen for fermentation. Keep the fermentation vessel and the bottle tightly closed.

Bottling

I recommend using a 1-quart (1 liter) sturdy glass bottle with a narrow neck and a tight-fitting lid (similar to a champagne bottle) as this shape will encourage carbonation to develop. The lid needs a good seal so that the fizz stays in the bottle. A bottle with a flip-top rubber stopper is suitable. You will also need a funnel.

Yeast strands

Strands and floaty bits may appear during the first fermentation stage as the wild yeasts gather in the mead. These are harmless and you can drink them or remove them by straining the mead.

Sediment

Some sediment (called "lees") may appear in both the first and second fermentation stages. This is normal. Either stir it up and add it to the finished mead, or strain it out and discard it when you bottle or serve the mead.

HOW TO KNOW WHEN YOUR
HONEY MEAD
IS READY FOR BOTTLING

SMELL
The mead should have an alcoholic, vinegary smell – it won't have a sweet, honey smell but will be a little more acidic. You will definitely notice a change from sweet to sour. If this has not yet happened, stir well and leave the mead to ferment for longer. I prefer to drink mead that is on the sweeter side.

LOOK
You should see small bubbles on the side of the fermentation vessel. You may see bubbles rising up from the bottom of the jar. There could also be bubbles at the top of the mead.

LISTEN
Honey mead is generally an active fermentation, so you should be able to hear the fermentation ticking along with the sound of fizzing and hissing.

TASTE
This is a full-bodied, warming and sometimes intense elixir. The flavor is aromatic and fills the mouth, and the taste is almost marshmallowy with its softness and sweetness.

TROUBLESHOOTING

WHAT IF THE BREW TURNS MOLDY?

If mold appears on the surface of the mead or any added ingredients, I advise you to discard the brew and start again.

WHAT IF THE BREW ISN'T FERMENTING?

If the brew isn't showing any signs of active fermentation, consider the following questions.

* **Have you been vigorously stirring the mead every day to encourage yeast activity?** If not, try stirring the mead a couple of times each day.
* **Did you use pasteurized honey?** If so, the brew may not ferment.
* **Is it too cold, perhaps in autumn or winter?** If so, leave it to ferment for longer.

WHAT IF FERMENTATION HAS STOPPED?

If the mead seems to have stopped fermenting, aerating it really well by stirring it to give the yeasts some oxygen should fix the issue. Temperature also plays an important part in successful fermentation – a hotter temperature will hasten fermentation, while cooler temperatures will slow fermentation time. If it's cold and the fermentation seems to have stopped, it could be because it's too cold for vigorous fermentation. You can buy heat mats from home brew shops if you want to keep the heat steady.

WHY DID MY HONEY MEAD TURN VISCOUS?

Generally this happens if the ratio of yeast to sugar to water is out of balance or if the mead has not been stirred often enough. Stir or shake the mead daily during the first 1 to 2 weeks of fermentation to activate the wild yeasts.

WHAT IF MY MEAD LOOKS CLOUDY AND THERE APPEARS TO BE SEDIMENT?

This can happen during active fermentation, and is generally nothing to worry about. The cloudiness shouldn't affect the taste and will settle out (clarify) as the mead continues to ferment. When you bottle your mead, it's preferable to filter out this sediment using a fine-mesh strainer.

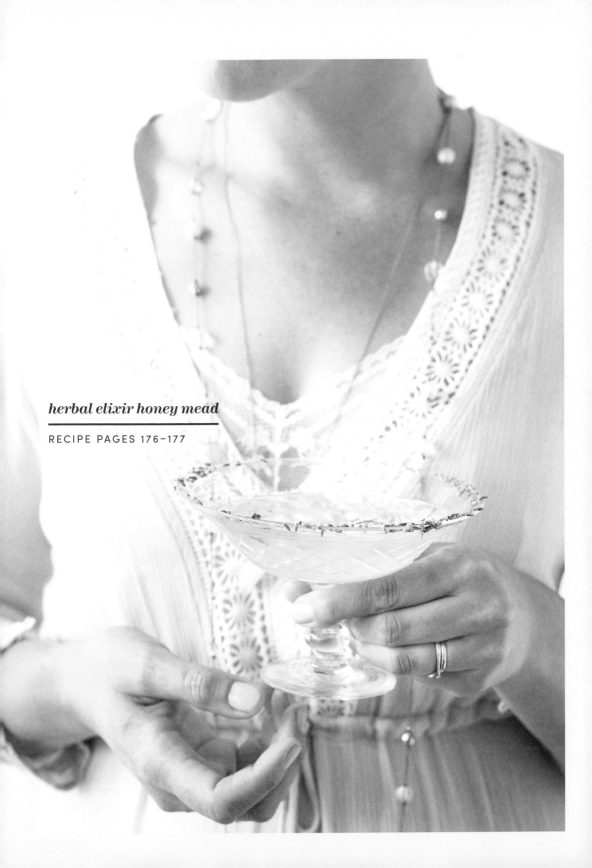

herbal elixir honey mead

RECIPE PAGES 176–177

RECIPES

basic honey mead

One of the main reasons I love honey is the amazing process of bees alchemizing nectar from flowers into honey. Honey mead is delicious and makes an easy, unique gift to give to a friend or loved one. I like to drink mead in a champagne flute because it amplifies the beauty of the natural fizz and feels so special.

Preparation time: 10 minutes **Fermentation time:** 1–6 weeks **Difficulty:** Easy
Shelf life: Refrigerate for up to 2 years **Makes:** About 1 quart (1 liter)

INGREDIENTS
1 cup (350 g) raw honey
1 quart (1 liter) filtered water or
   spring water

PRIMARY FERMENTATION
Put the honey into a 1-quart (1 liter) wide-mouth glass jar with a lid and add 1¼ cups (300 ml) of the filtered water. Mix well to dissolve the honey. Tightly seal the jar and then shake vigorously.

Add enough of the remaining filtered water to make up 1 quart (1 liter), tightly seal the jar and shake vigorously.

Place the jar in a cool, dark place. Give the mixture a vigorous shake or stir every day, if you can. After 1 week you should start to see bubbles forming – this is the yeasts waking up. Taste the mead; if it's still too sweet ("young") put the lid back on and leave it to ferment for longer. Skim any scum off the surface using a fine-mesh strainer.

Continue to shake or stir the mead daily, and taste it every week or so. Once it's slightly sour and fizzy, it's ready to bottle. This could take anywhere from 1 week to several months, depending on your taste and the temperature. As a general rule, I leave mead to ferment for around 1 month.

BOTTLING

Put a funnel in the opening of a 1-quart (1 liter) glass bottle with a tight-fitting lid. Slowly pour the honey mead into the bottle and tightly seal the bottle lid.

SECONDARY FERMENTATION

If you are satisfied with the taste and level of carbonation, store the honey mead in the fridge, and enjoy cold or at room temperature.

Otherwise, leave the mead on the counter to allow the carbonation to build further for 2 to 7 days. Don't "burp" it as you want the carbonation to build.

DRINK UP

When the honey mead is as fizzy as you like, store it in the fridge to slow the fermentation process, and enjoy cold or at room temperature.

If you want more fizz and more sweetness, add another tablespoon or so of honey, tightly seal the bottle lid and shake vigorously. Leave the mead on the counter to ferment for 2 to 7 days more, or until as fizzy as you like, then store in the fridge.

winter spice honey mead with nutmeg and clove

The fire is on, you are curled up in a cashmere blanket with a good book or your favorite magazine and a warming glass of spicy honey mead is at your side – a perfect winter evening. You can add a strip of orange zest when you're bottling the mead to give the mead a citrus flavor.

Preparation time: 10 minutes **Fermentation time:** 1–6 weeks **Difficulty:** Easy
Shelf life: Refrigerate for up to 2 years **Makes:** About 1 quart (1 liter)

INGREDIENTS

1 recipe basic honey mead
  (page 172)
pinch of freshly grated nutmeg
1 clove

PRIMARY FERMENTATION

Follow the instructions for basic honey mead, adding the nutmeg and clove once the honey has dissolved.

BOTTLING

Follow the instructions for basic honey mead.

SECONDARY FERMENTATION

If you are satisfied with the taste and level of carbonation, store the honey mead in the fridge, and enjoy cold or at room temperature.

Otherwise, leave the mead on the counter to allow the carbonation to build further for 2 to 7 days. Don't "burp" it as you want the carbonation to build.

DRINK UP

When the honey mead is as fizzy as you like, store it in the fridge to slow the fermentation process, and enjoy cold or at room temperature.

If you want more fizz and more sweetness, add another tablespoon or so of honey, tightly seal the bottle lid and shake vigorously. Leave the mead on the counter to ferment for 2 to 7 days more, or until as fizzy as you like, then store in the fridge.

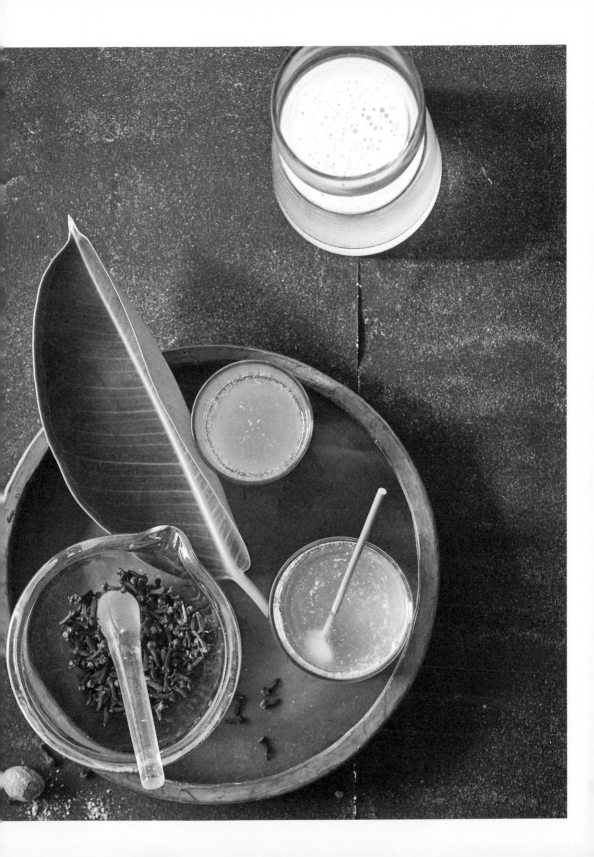

herbal elixir honey mead

Lavender is traditionally used to calm the nervous system. I use lavender oil every day on my wrists and in an oil burner on my desk, and every night I add a few drops to my daughters' pillows to help ease them into a calm and relaxed state for a peaceful night's sleep. In this herbal elixir, we preserve and bottle the medicinal qualities of the lavender in the honey mead. Use unsprayed lavender sprigs from your own garden or neighborhood. You can also buy dried lavender through some online stores, and some supermarkets and health food stores sell lavender sprigs in the fresh herb section.

Preparation time: 10 minutes **Fermentation time:** 1–6 weeks **Difficulty:** Easy
Shelf life: Refrigerate for up to 2 years **Makes:** About 1 quart (1 liter)

INGREDIENTS

1 recipe basic honey mead (page 172)
2 or 3 unsprayed lavender sprigs, plus 1 extra sprig (optional)

(See recipe photo on page 171.)

PRIMARY FERMENTATION
Follow the instructions for basic honey mead, adding the lavender sprigs once the honey has dissolved.

BOTTLING
Put a funnel in the opening of a 1-quart (1 liter) glass bottle with a tight-fitting lid. Scoop out and discard the lavender sprigs. Slowly pour the honey mead into the bottle. Add the extra lavender sprig, if using, and tightly seal the bottle lid.

SECONDARY FERMENTATION
If you are satisfied with the taste and level of carbonation, store the honey mead in the fridge, and enjoy cold or at room temperature.

Otherwise, leave the mead on the counter to allow the carbonation to build further for 2 to 7 days. Don't "burp" it as you want the carbonation to build.

DRINK UP

When the honey mead is as fizzy as you like, store it in the fridge to slow the fermentation process, and enjoy cold or at room temperature.

If you want more fizz and more sweetness, add another tablespoon or so of honey, tightly seal the bottle lid and shake vigorously. Leave the mead on the counter to ferment for 2 to 7 days more, or until as fizzy as you like, then store in the fridge.

——

TIPS *You can also cover the lavender with hot water and leave it to cool to room temperature, then strain the lavender water and add it to the honey and water mixture in the primary fermentation stage.*

Use any herb you like, such as dandelion, rosemary, pineapple sage, chaga, mint or chamomile.

——

rosewater honey mead

The cultivation of roses for medicinal and culinary means has been in use since the Persian era. This mead is a gorgeous and decadent ferment that would traditionally be considered a "rhodomel" mead as it's derived from roses. You can use either rosebuds, rose petals, rosewater, rose essential oil or rosehip tea bags to impart the rose flavor – see the variations at the end of the recipe.

Preparation time: 10 minutes **Fermentation time:** 1–6 weeks **Difficulty:** Easy
Shelf life: Refrigerate for up to 2 years **Makes:** About 1 quart (1 liter)

INGREDIENTS

4 to 6 edible organic unsprayed rosebuds or rose petals, plus extra 4 rosebuds (optional)
1 cup (350 g) raw honey
1 quart (1 liter) filtered water or spring water

PRIMARY FERMENTATION

Add the rosebuds or rose petals to a mug and cover with ½ cup (100 ml) boiling water. Leave to cool to room temperature. Remove and discard the rosebuds or petals.

Pour the honey and rosewater into a 1-quart (1 liter) wide-mouth glass jar with a lid and add 1¼ cups (300 ml) of the filtered water. Follow the remaining primary fermentation instructions for basic honey mead.

BOTTLING

Follow the instructions for basic honey mead, adding the extra rosebuds, if using, before you seal the bottle.

SECONDARY FERMENTATION

If you are satisfied with the taste and level of carbonation, store the honey mead in the fridge, and enjoy cold or at room temperature.

Otherwise, leave the mead on the counter to allow the carbonation to build further for 2 to 7 days. Don't "burp" it as you want the carbonation to build.

DRINK UP

When the honey mead is as fizzy as you like, store it in the fridge to slow the fermentation process, and enjoy cold or at room temperature.

If you want more fizz and more sweetness, add another tablespoon or so of honey, tightly seal the bottle lid and shake vigorously. Leave the mead on the counter to ferment for 2 to 7 days more, or until as fizzy as you like, then store in the fridge.

TIP *Add some edible dried rose petals or rose-flavored cotton candy to the glass when serving the mead.*

VARIATIONS
Instead of steeping the rosebuds or rose petals and adding them with the honey, choose one of the following options.

Rosewater
Add 2 tablespoons to ¼ cup (60 ml) rosewater when bottling the honey mead. Rosewater varies in strength, so add a little at a time, tasting as you go. You can also add 4 edible rosebuds to the honey mead to add more flavor and to add a pretty touch.

Rose essential oil
Add 1 or 2 drops of edible pure rose essential oil when bottling the honey mead. Pure essential oil is incredibly concentrated, so you'll only need a small amount. Add the first drop, taste and then add a second drop if needed. You can also add 4 edible rosebuds to the honey mead at this stage.

Rose petals
Add a handful of edible fresh or dried organic rose petals to the jar with the honey and water before the initial fermentation stage. Remove or retain the rose petals when you bottle the honey mead.

Rosehip tea
Use 4 rosehip tea bags and 2 cups (500 ml) boiling water to brew some rosehip tea. Add this rosehip tea to the honey water before the initial fermentation stage. You will need to use a strainer when bottling the honey mead, as quite a lot of sediment remains.

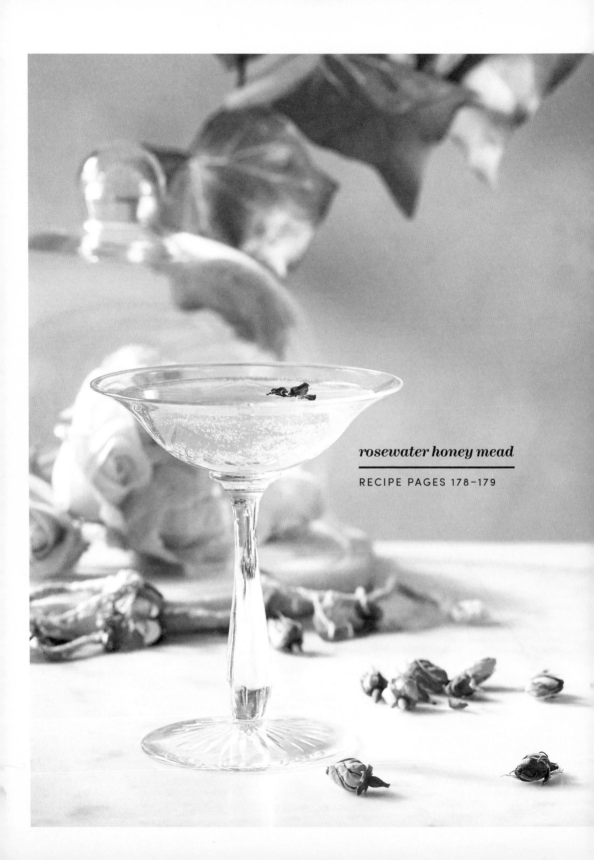

rosewater honey mead

RECIPE PAGES 178–179

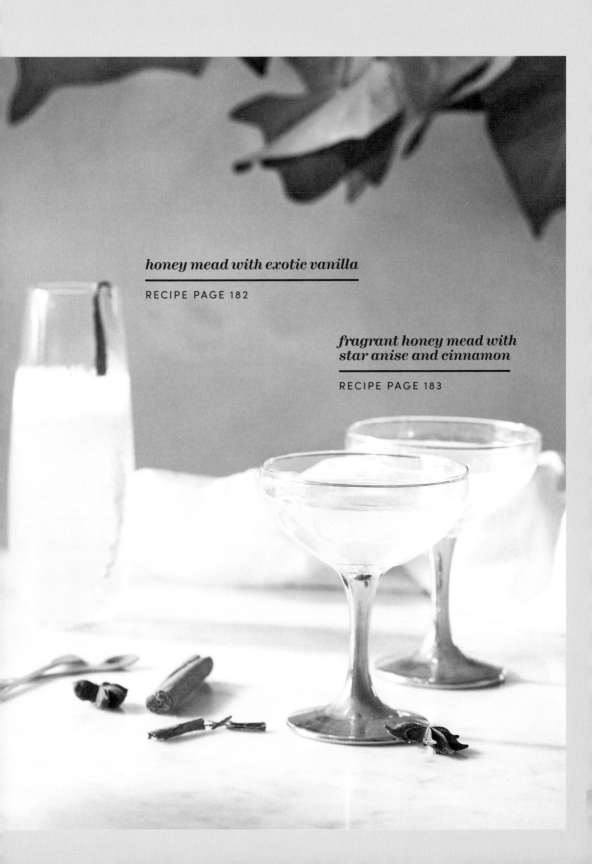

honey mead with exotic vanilla

RECIPE PAGE 182

*fragrant honey mead with
star anise and cinnamon*

RECIPE PAGE 183

honey mead with exotic vanilla

Vanilla beans are the fermented and dried seedpods of a tropical climbing orchid, *Vanilla planifolia*, that is native to the tropical rain forests of Central America. The Mayans used this highly prized bean to flavor their cacao drinks. The creamy notes of vanilla pair stunningly with the honey in the mead. This type of mead would be classified as "metheglin" (medicine).

Preparation time: 10 minutes **Fermentation time:** 1–6 weeks **Difficulty:** Easy
Shelf life: Refrigerate for up to 2 years **Makes:** About 1 quart (1 liter)

INGREDIENTS
1 recipe basic honey mead
    (page 172)
1 vanilla bean

PRIMARY FERMENTATION
Follow the instructions for basic honey mead.

BOTTLING
Follow the instructions for basic honey mead, adding the vanilla bean before you seal the bottle.

SECONDARY FERMENTATION
If you are satisfied with the taste and level of carbonation, store the honey mead in the fridge, and enjoy cold or at room temperature.

Otherwise, leave the mead on the counter to allow the carbonation to build further for 2 to 7 days. Don't "burp" it as you want the carbonation to build.

DRINK UP
When the honey mead is as fizzy as you like, store it in the fridge to slow the fermentation process, and enjoy cold or at room temperature.

If you want more fizz and more sweetness, add another tablespoon or so of honey, tightly seal the bottle lid and shake vigorously. Leave the mead on the counter to ferment for 2 to 7 days more, or until as fizzy as you like, then store in the fridge.

fragrant honey mead with star anise and cinnamon

———

This is another variety of honey mead that would traditionally be classified as "metheglin" because of the addition of the spices. Star anise is a star-shaped spice with a licorice flavor and fragrance. It has medicinal and antioxidant properties and is known to be antifungal and antibacterial. Cinnamon is a beautiful warming spice that's cut from the inner bark of the cinnamon tree.

Preparation time: 10 minutes **Fermentation time:** 1–6 weeks **Difficulty:** Easy
Shelf life: Refrigerate for up to 2 years **Makes:** About 1 quart (1 liter)

———

INGREDIENTS
1 recipe basic honey mead
   (page 172)
1 cinnamon stick
1 star anise

PRIMARY FERMENTATION
Follow the instructions for basic honey mead.

BOTTLING
Follow the instructions for basic honey mead, adding the cinnamon stick and star anise before you seal the bottle.

SECONDARY FERMENTATION
If you are satisfied with the taste and level of carbonation, store the honey mead in the fridge, and enjoy cold or at room temperature.

Otherwise, leave the mead on the counter to allow the carbonation to build further for 2 to 7 days. Don't "burp" it as you want the carbonation to build.

DRINK UP
When the honey mead is as fizzy as you like, store it in the fridge to slow the fermentation process, and enjoy cold or at room temperature.

If you want more fizz and more sweetness, add another tablespoon or so of honey, tightly seal the bottle lid and shake vigorously. Leave the mead on the counter to ferment for 2 to 7 days more, or until as fizzy as you like, then store in the fridge.

GLOSSARY

Aerobic fermentation
This is the type of fermentation that requires oxygen. The fermentation vessel needs to be covered with a light covering, such as cheesecloth, and sealed with a rubber band so that pests can't get in. Examples of aerobic fermentation are water kefir, milk kefir, kombucha and Jun.

Anaerobic fermentation
This is the type of fermentation that doesn't require oxygen. The fermentation vessel needs to be tightly sealed with a lid so that no oxygen can get in, although during the first fermentation stage some oxygen is needed to activate the wild yeasts (see page 167). Examples of anaerobic fermentation are beet kvass and honey mead.

Antioxidant
Ingredients that prevent or reduce damage from free radicals.

Bacteria
Bacteria are single-celled organisms that can exist independently, cooperatively or parasitically. Fermentation relies on the bacteria working cooperatively.

Burping
This refers to the technique of slightly opening a lid or stopper on a bottle to release some pressure that may have built up during the secondary fermentation stage.

Culture/starter culture
This is the starting SCOBY or culture that is used to ferment the collection of ingredients in cultured fermentation.

First ferment/primary fermentation
This is the first stage of fermentation, which transforms the collection of ingredients into a more digestible form that is generally lower in sugar.

Milk kefir grains/culture/starter
This is the actual culture that you need to make milk kefir and it must be acquired from somewhere. The terms *grains*, *culture* and *starter* are generally interchangeable.

Mother
This is the name given to the kombucha SCOBY.

Natural carbonation
This is when fizz can develop (generally during and after secondary fermentation) as a result of the carbon dioxide that is produced during the fermentation process.

Prebiotics
Prebiotics are indigestible fiber that can pass through the intestine and serve as a food source for the probiotics and stimulate probiotic growth in the gastrointestinal tract.

Probiotics
Probiotics are beneficial bacteria and yeasts that, when taken in adequate amounts, offer health benefits.

SCOBY
An acronym for symbiotic colony of bacteria and yeast, SCOBY is the name generally given to a kombucha culture. However, it can also be used to refer to water kefir grains, Jun culture and some other cultures.

Second ferment/secondary fermentation
The second stage of fermentation is generally where flavoring ingredients are added and when carbonation is allowed to naturally build in the bottle.

Water kefir grains/culture/starter
This is the actual culture that you need to make water kefir and it must be acquired from somewhere. The terms *grains*, *culture* and *starter* are generally interchangeable.

Wild fermentation
This type of fermentation does not rely on a starter culture; rather, it relies on the naturally occurring yeasts and bacteria that live on the surface of ingredients and in the air. This type of fermentation can be spontaneous, but it can also be helped along by stirring, shaking and aerating.

Yeasts
These are fungi that can convert sugars into alcohol.

INDEX

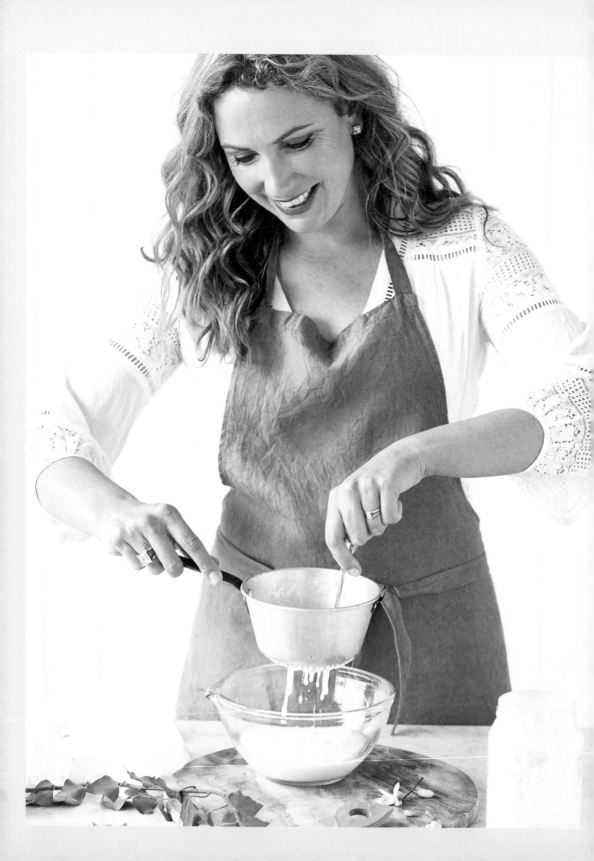

ACKNOWLEDGMENTS

I'd love to pay my respects to our ancestors who understood how to harness fermentation for better health and harvest preservation. Their knowledge and cultivation of these cultures and processes is valuable beyond measure.

I wrote this book for you, the reader. Thank you for trusting me to guide you through the exciting journey of fermentation.

Thank you to my community of recipe testers who joined in the adventure.

Massive thanks to Jody Scott who believed in me from our first water kefir date. You have a beautiful generous spirit, and I'm forever grateful to you.

Jane Morrow, Emma Hutchinson, Megan Pigott, Justine Harding, Sarah Odgers and the entire team at Murdoch Books, thank you for your guidance and dedication to this project.

My steadfast husband for your incredible support and wisdom, and for being my unwavering rock.

My divine children through whom I see the whole world. You are the compass directing me to become a more gracious person, and you make me believe that angels do indeed live on Earth.

To my family who have encouraged and believed in me, thank you.

ABOUT THE AUTHOR

Felicity Evans is the alchemist and founder at Imbibe Living. Her company crafts a range of sparkling probiotic water kefirs and offers cultures on the website imbibeliving.com. She's created an online course providing you the tools and techniques to confidently ferment your own probiotic drinks at home.

Originally published as *Probiotic Drinks at Home* by Murdoch Books in Australia in 2017 and in the UK in 2018.
First published in North America by The Experiment, LLC, in 2018.

The Experiment, LLC
220 East 23rd Street, Suite 600
New York, NY 10010-4674
theexperimentpublishing.com

This book contains the opinions and ideas of its author. It is intended to provide helpful and informative material on the subjects addressed in the book. It is sold with the understanding that the author and publisher are not engaged in rendering medical, health, or any other kind of personal professional services in the book. The author and publisher specifically disclaim all responsibility for any liability, loss, or risk—personal or otherwise—that is incurred as a consequence, directly or indirectly, of the use and application of any of the contents of this book.

Many of the designations used by manufacturers and sellers to distinguish their products are claimed as trademarks. Where those designations appear in this book and The Experiment was aware of a trademark claim, the designations have been capitalized.

The Experiment's books are available at special discounts when purchased in bulk for premiums and sales promotions as well as for fund-raising or educational use. For details, contact us at info@theexperimentpublishing.com.

Library of Congress Cataloging-in-Publication Data available upon request

ISBN 978-1-61519-448-3
Ebook ISBN 978-1-61519-449-0

Cover design by Sarah Smith
Text design by Murdoch Books
Cover photographs by Rob Palmer

Manufactured in China
Distributed by Workman Publishing Company, Inc.
Distributed simultaneously in Canada by the University of Toronto Press

First printing March 2018
10 9 8 7 6 5 4 3 2 1

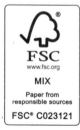

FSC
www.fsc.org
MIX
Paper from
responsible sources
FSC® C023121